CLINICIAN'S GUIDE TO RESEARCH
METHODS IN FAMILY THERAPY

Also available

Essential Assessment Skills for Couple and Family Therapists
Lee Williams, Todd M. Edwards, JoEllen Patterson, and Larry Chamow

Essential Skills in Family Therapy, Second Edition:
From the First Interview to Termination
JoEllen Patterson, Lee Williams, Todd M. Edwards,
Larry Chamow, and Claudia Grauf-Grounds

The Therapist's Guide to Psychopharmacology, Revised Edition:
Working with Patients, Families, and Physicians to Optimize Care
JoEllen Patterson, A. Ari Albala,
Margaret E. McCahill, and Todd M. Edwards

CLINICIAN'S GUIDE TO RESEARCH METHODS IN FAMILY THERAPY

Foundations of Evidence-Based Practice

Lee Williams
JoEllen Patterson
Todd M. Edwards

THE GUILFORD PRESS
New York   London

Copyright © 2014 The Guilford Press
A Division of Guilford Publications, Inc.
370 Seventh Avenue, Suite 1200, New York, NY 10001
www.guilford.com

Paperback edition 2018

Printed in the United States of America

This book is printed on acid-free paper.

Last digit is print number: 9   8   7   6   5   4   3

The authors have checked with sources believed to be reliable in their efforts to provide
information that is complete and generally in accord with the standards of practice that
are accepted at the time of publication. However, in view of the possibility of human error
or changes in behavioral, mental health, or medical sciences, neither the author, nor the
editor and publisher, nor any other party who has been involved in the preparation or
publication of this work warrants that the information contained herein is in every respect
accurate or complete, and they are not responsible for any errors or omissions or the
results obtained from the use of such information. Readers are encouraged to confirm the
information contained in this book with other sources.

Library of Congress Cataloging-in-Publication Data

Williams, Lee LMFT.
  Clinician's guide to research methods in family therapy : Foundations of evidence-based
practice / Lee Williams, JoEllen Patterson, Todd M. Edwards.
     pages cm
  Includes bibliographical references and index.
  ISBN 978-1-4625-1597-4 (hardback : acid-free paper)
  ISBN 978-1-4625-3606-1 (paperback : acid-free paper)
  1. Family psychotherapy—Methodology.   2. Family psychotherapy—Research.
3. Couples therapy.   I. Patterson, JoEllen.   II. Edwards, Todd M.   III. Title.
  RC488.5W5617 2014
  616.89′156—dc23
                                                                              2014006716

About the Authors

Lee Williams, PhD, is Professor in the Marital and Family Therapy Program at the University of San Diego. His research interests include family therapy training, marriage preparation, and couples with religious differences. Dr. Williams is coauthor of *Essential Skills in Family Therapy, Second Edition,* and *Essential Assessment Skills for Couple and Family Therapists.*

JoEllen Patterson, PhD, is Professor in the Marital and Family Therapy Program at the University of San Diego. She is also a voluntary Clinical Associate Professor in the Divisions of Family Medicine and Global Health as well as the Department of Psychiatry at the University of California, San Diego, School of Medicine. Dr. Patterson has published five books and numerous articles. She is coauthor of *Essential Assessment Skills for Couple and Family Therapists; Essential Skills in Family Therapy, Second Edition,* and *The Therapist's Guide to Psychopharmacology, Revised Edition.* Dr. Patterson serves on the editorial boards of *Families, Systems, and Health* and the *Journal of Marital and Family Therapy.* Her Fulbright Scholarships have allowed her to work in Norway, New Zealand, Hong Kong, and elsewhere.

Todd M. Edwards, PhD, is Professor and Director of the Marital and Family Therapy Program at the University of San Diego, and provides individual and family therapy in the Division of Family Medicine at the University of California, San Diego, School of Medicine. His research and teaching interests focus on the integration of family-oriented mental health services into primary care settings; family therapy training; and male friendship in adulthood. He is Associate Editor of *Families, Systems, and Health.*

Preface

One of the challenges we have faced in the master's training program for family therapy that we teach is engendering in students an appreciation of the value of research in informing their clinical work. Students typically enjoy many of the courses we offer in our program, such as those on family therapy theories and psychopathology. However, students are frequently less enthusiastic about the research methods class we require them to take.

Traditionally, whoever taught the class in our program faced many of the same challenges instructors in other training programs encounter. First, students would come into our program with varying levels of expertise in research. Some of our students who had earned undergraduate degrees in psychology had taken multiple research courses, and may even have had experience in a research lab. Other students came from disciplines like English, fashion design, and music, which provided them with little or no exposure to research.

Second, students would often experience initial anxiety about learning and mastering research concepts. For many, this anxiety seemed rooted in their lack of confidence in their mathematical abilities. These students would equate research with statistics, which was then equated with mathematics. This misconception about research, coupled with the anxiety it generated, led some students to distance themselves from research, rather than embrace it.

Anxiety about learning research was not necessarily restricted to those who were taking the research course for the first time. Many students confessed that they had forgotten what they had learned from earlier courses, with the unstated implication that what they had learned before was not worth remembering. Learning (and retaining) research concepts was important if you were going to do research, but how important was it to someone who wanted to be a clinician? Thus, learning research did not seem to resonate with these students' emerging identities as therapists or clinicians.

This book has emerged out of our struggle to make our research class relevant to our students. When the course was first taught in our program, it followed a traditional research methods curriculum. The primary focus was on teaching students about various research designs and statistics. Understandably, our students sometimes had a difficult time seeing the connection between the concepts they were learning in class and the work they were doing with clients in the therapy room.

Over time the course evolved, and we began to make explicit that its goal was to teach our students to be effective consumers of research, and not necessarily to turn them into researchers (although some were interested in this path). This shift helped to shape the focus of the course to some extent, but it still largely focused on the mechanics of research rather than its application.

Around this time, we began writing articles on evidence-based practice in family therapy. The first article (Patterson, Miller, Carnes, & Wilson, 2004) described the potential for evidence-based ideas to be applied to family therapy. The next article (Williams, Patterson, & Miller, 2006) built on the initial article, but offered more practical guidance on the steps therapists could take to implement evidence-based practice in their clinical work.

These articles marked an important transition in how we taught the class, as we began to integrate evidence-based practice into the instruction. For example, the second article became a required reading, and we assigned a project in which the students applied research findings to a clinical vignette that they selected. This exercise gave them the opportunity to experiment with using research findings in an applied way.

We eventually decided that we needed to go farther in promoting evidence-based practice in the class. We believed this would reinforce the connection between research and clinical work, and might serve to motivate our students to learn research.

However, we did not feel there was a book that captured how we wanted to teach the course. We wanted a book that would provide the fundamentals of research so our students could become knowledgeable consumers of reports on experiments, surveys, and so forth. Yet, we did not want a traditional textbook that focused only on research designs and statistics. We also wanted a book that addressed the clinical complexities therapists encounter as they try to apply research to their work with clients. We sought a book that covered both fundamental research concepts and evidence-based practice, and with content that could be reasonably covered in a single semester. Because we could not find such a book, we decided to write it.

The first chapter of this book argues why learning research can be valuable. It also attempts to challenge some of the misconceptions many students have about research, which can interfere with their motivation to learn research. After this introductory chapter, the first half of the book is devoted to the fundamentals of research designs and statistics. This part of the book captures our best thinking on how to make research concepts interesting and easily understood. Our goal has been to describe research in a simple and relatable way, much as we have done with our other books on family therapy skills (Patterson, Williams, Edwards, Chamow, & Grauf-Grounds, 2009), psychopharmacology (Patterson, Albala, McCahill, & Edwards, 2010), and assessment (Williams, Edwards, Patterson, & Chamow, 2011). We also show how research concepts often parallel concepts in the clinical world, although they sometimes seem disconnected because of the different terms used.

The second half of the book focuses on evidence-based practice. As in the first half of the book, we attempt to write about the ideas in a simple and accessible manner. Yet, at the same time, we speak plainly about the challenges therapists may encounter in applying research to clinical practice. We offer guidance to therapists on how to navigate these challenges.

Despite the hurdles therapists can face in applying research, we earnestly believe the struggle is worth it. Accessing knowledge through the research literature can add to and enhance the clinical knowledge we already possess. Knowledge from research and our clinical experience, coupled with our compassion for our clients, can help us be effective therapists.

LEE WILLIAMS
JOELLEN PATTERSON
TODD EDWARDS
University of San Diego

Acknowledgments

We would like to thank Jenee James for her contributions to Chapters 15 and 17, and Rose Schafer and Joe Scherger for their contributions to Chapter 19. In addition, we would like to thank Rose Schafer and Samantha Hoffman for their assistance in preparing the Glossary. Finally, we would like to express our appreciation to the following individuals who provided helpful feedback on the book chapters (in alphabetical order): Fred Galloway, Samantha Hoffman, Julie Melekian, Evelyn Robarts, Anastacia Tobin, and Laura Weese.

Contents

CHAPTER 1

Learning to Apply Research

Why Bother?

Susan is a beginning therapist working with the Robinson family. The family is seeking treatment because Michael, who is 14, was caught shoplifting. Susan feels like the family is challenging and resistant to her suggestions for change. In class, Susan reads a qualitative study that describes how families being treated for adolescent drug abuse experience family therapy (Kuehl, Newfield, & Joanning, 1990). In their discussion of the results, the researchers commented that families could encounter "therapist resistance," which occurs when therapists become insistent in promoting their agenda for therapy despite the family's reservations. After reading this article, Susan began to wonder if she is exhibiting therapist resistance. In her next session, Susan spends more time joining with the family and asking how they thought therapy should proceed. After this session, Susan begins to reformulate an approach that is more consistent with the family's view of the problem. She soon discovers that movement is beginning to happen in therapy.

Susan's experience illustrates the power of research to inform and improve our therapy. Unfortunately, many clinicians do not take full advantage of the benefits research has to offer. One reason for this is that many therapists are not taught the required skills for using research clinically. Their introduction to research typically focuses on research designs and statistics, with little or no instruction on how these concepts might be applied clinically. Although a basic knowledge of research designs and statistics is necessary, it is often not sufficient if one is going to take the next step and use research to inform one's clinical work. Therefore, our goal in writing this book is twofold. First, we want to provide you with the essential knowledge of research that you will need as a clinician. Second, and equally important, we want to give you the skills you need to apply research clinically through evidence-based practice. Both are necessary if you are going to realize the full potential that research has to offer for enhancing your clinical effectiveness. Before describing the book in more detail, let us explore in more depth why applying research to clinical work can be valuable.

WHAT IS RESEARCH (AND WHY SHOULD I CARE)?

Do you want to be the most effective practitioner you can be? If you answered yes, then you will be interested in learning how to apply research to your clinical work. At its most basic level, research is simply about gaining knowledge. Figure 1.1 shows the multiple ways we can acquire clinical knowledge, which includes learning from theory, supervision, life experience, and clinical experience. This book will teach you how to use research to enhance your clinical knowledge.

In a press conference during the war with Iraq, Secretary of Defense Donald Rumsfeld stated, "There are known knowns. These are things we know that we know. There are known unknowns. That is to say, there are things that we know we don't know. But there are also unknown unknowns. There are things we don't know we don't know." This quote suggests the different ways that research can inform our knowledge (Williams, Patterson, & Miller, 2006).

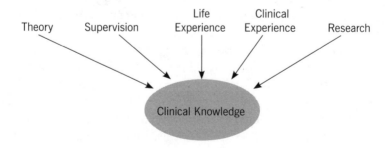

FIGURE 1.1. Sources of clinical knowledge.

First, research can confirm our known knowns. In other words, it can help us confirm something that we suspect is true based on knowledge we have gained through clinical or life experience. When Cassandra read about emotionally focused therapy, she found that it deeply resonated with how she worked with couples. When she discovered that it was an empirically supported treatment, she had greater confidence in her approach with couples.

Second, research can help us learn something we don't know. Research can help you answer the known unknowns in your clinical work. Nyesha was recently assigned Owen, a 14-year-old boy with a diagnosis of autism spectrum disorder. Recognizing her lack of knowledge regarding Owen's disorder, Nyesha reviewed some of the empirical research on treating autism spectrum disorder. She learned the importance of strengthening social skills in treating this disorder and incorporated this information into her treatment with Owen.

Third, research can help us identify what we don't know. It is not uncommon for research to raise new questions in addition to providing new insights. As a result, research can sometimes illuminate what we don't know. Therapists can experience this same phenomenon in their clinical work. Isabella was fairly confident that she could help a recently engaged couple address problems in their relationship. Eve had discovered from a friend that Dominic had bought an engagement ring several months before, but never proposed to her. Eve referred back to this several times when discussing her concerns in therapy. During the course of treatment, Isabella read an article by Johnson, Makinen, and Millikin (2001) that studied treatment failures in emotionally focused therapy. In analyzing these treatment failures, the authors frequently found an event that the couple seemed to have difficulty getting past, which the authors labeled as an attachment injury. Isabella recognized that Eve's discovery of the ring and Dominic's failure to propose had created an attachment injury for her. Isabella was unaware of attachment injuries prior to reading this article, one of her unknown unknowns. Using the model proposed in the article, Isabella helped the couple work through the attachment injury, which led to a successful outcome in therapy. This experience reinforced for Isabella the need to read research to expand her knowledge, including learning about things of which she was unaware.

However, research can be invaluable in a fourth way that is not evident from the Rumsfeld quote. Research can also disconfirm something that we believe to be true. As a beginning therapist, Ricardo believed that if you helped couples reduce conflict in their relationship, they would automatically become closer. However, research by Gottman and Gottman (2008) suggests that developing positive behaviors and reducing conflict seemed to be governed by different processes. This helped Ricardo recognize that a different set of interventions was necessary to build a couple's closeness beyond just reducing conflict.

Beyond these general ways of adding to our knowledge, research can inform assessment and treatment in more specific ways (Williams et al., 2006). First, research can help us better understand our client's experiences, which may be particularly helpful if we have not had a similar experience. Even if we have had something similar happen to us, our reaction may have been quite different from our client's. Knowing the research may teach us not to assume that our experience is the same as our client's. Qualitative research can be particularly useful in providing a description of how clients experience certain phenomena. For example, one qualitative study provided a rich description of how clients responded to the disclosure of an affair (Olson, Russell, Higgins-Kessler, & Miller, 2002). Having a better understanding of our client's experiences through research will enhance our assessment, joining, and credibility.

Second, research can help guide our assessment by informing us of important factors that are related to disorders or problems we encounter in therapy. Poor family conflict management, poor parental monitoring, caregiver psychopathology and drug abuse, association with deviant peers, and poor socialization skills are among the many factors that research has indicated are related to conduct disorder in youth (Henggeler & Sheidow, 2003). Therefore, these would be important areas to assess when addressing youth with this diagnosis.

Third, instruments developed for research purposes may be useful in clinical assessment. A classic example is the Dyadic Adjustment Scale (Spanier, 1976), which is a widely used instrument in research for measuring marital adjustment. The Dyadic Adjustment Scale has also been used extensively in clinical settings to assess relationship or marital quality among couples.

Fourth, research can inform which treatment approach will be effective with a particular problem. For example, a therapist who works with couples in marital distress may choose to use one of the empirically supported treatments for couple therapy such as emotionally focused therapy or behavioral couple therapy (Johnson, 2003). We will discuss the use of empirically supported treatments in therapy in greater detail in Chapter 16.

Fifth, research can also help identify which elements of a treatment are important to its success. Common factors may emerge when comparing the results of different kinds of treatment. For example, several clinical researchers who have developed family-based treatments for schizophrenia reached a consensus on treatment principles that can guide therapists working with families with a member who has schizophrenia (McFarlane, Dixon, Lukens, & Luckstead, 2003). Process research (see Chapter 7) can also help us identify the key ingredients to bring about change. For example, one study demonstrated that softening events are associated with positive outcomes in emotionally focused therapy (Johnson & Greenberg, 1988).

One could argue that enhancing our clinical knowledge through research is an ethical responsibility. When we seek treatment from a medical professional, we certainly hope the physician has the latest knowledge regarding the most effective treatments for our particular illness or problem. Should our clients expect anything less from us? Becoming a skilled consumer of research is one of the best ways of making sure we can offer our clients the most effective treatments.

WE ARE ALL RESEARCHERS

If research is viewed as a means of acquiring knowledge, then we all could be considered researchers. In fact, we begin life as researchers:

> "Babies are very good at tracking statistical information in their environment," says Laura Schulz, a professor of brain and cognitive sciences at M.I.T. "They're incredibly sensitive to human action and intentional acts in the world. They watch what people are doing to learn causal connections." Babies will grab the same object over and over, replicating experiences, testing them out, conducting their own experiments. If I smile, will Mommy smile back? (Paul, 2006)

We don't stop learning as infants, but continue to grow and learn throughout our life.

Practicing therapy is a lot like doing research when viewed from this perspective. We make careful observations of our clients, develop hypotheses, and conduct interventions based on our hypotheses. The results from our interventions (experiments) help us confirm or disconfirm our hypotheses. We take what we have learned from one client and try to discern through repetition whether our knowledge generalizes to other clients. There are also strong parallels between how qualitative researchers conduct their work and how clinicians do therapy (which we will discuss in Chapter 6). Indeed, the parallels are so strong that participants in qualitative studies can experience therapeutic benefits (Drury, Francis, & Chapman, 2007; McCoyd & Shdaimah, 2007; Murray, 2003; Shamai, 2003)!

Unfortunately, we are prone to making several mistakes in our normal, everyday pursuit of knowledge (Babbie, 2007). What makes "researchers" different from us is that they follow a rigorous set of principles when attempting to acquire knowledge. By following the scientific principles described below, researchers hope to avoid these common mistakes.

The first principle researchers follow is to make careful observations or measurements. For example, researchers may use audio or video recordings of interactions so that they can review and accurately measure what is happening in them. In our everyday life, we generally are not careful observers. We are also vulnerable to selective observation, where we pay attention only to things that are consistent with what we believe. During the course of therapy, one woman ignored her husband's efforts to change. Instead, she focused only on his shortcomings because she was convinced she had made a mistake in marrying him.

Confirming a cause and effect relationship by carefully ruling out competing explanations for why something happens is a second important scientific principle. Researchers refer to this as **internal validity**, and rely primarily on research designs (e.g., experiments) to establish cause and effect. We are also interested in identifying the underlying causes to events in our lives, but we may not be as careful as researchers in considering alternative explanations. A therapist doing bereavement counseling may be quick to assume that his client's progress is due to therapy. However, it is possible that the client's grief improved through a natural mourning process that occurred over time.

A number of factors may make us vulnerable to drawing inaccurate inferences about cause and effect in our daily lives. Sometimes we use rationalizations to protect our ego. For example, rather than admit to his own possible shortcomings, Eric assumed he was passed over for a promotion because his boss favored another employee. We may also fall victim to illogical reasoning. One example is the gambler's fallacy, where a string of bad or good luck is thought to predict the opposite outcome. We may also attribute supernatural or mystical causes to events that we do not understand. After her husband's heart attack, Carol could not comprehend why he died so unexpectedly. Carol concluded God must have been punishing her for the sexual abuse she suffered as a child.

The third principle researchers follow is being careful about how far they generalize their conclusions based on the data or information they have collected. Researchers refer to this as **external validity**. External validity is largely determined by how representative our sample is relative to the people or phenomenon to which we want to generalize. In our personal lives, we may be too quick to overgeneralize. We may assume something is true in general when it is true for only a specific set of people or circumstances. Arturo and his wife Hazel came to therapy because of trust issues. Hazel was tired of Arturo's accusations that she was being unfaithful, which she denied. She believed Arturo's lack of trust stemmed from his fear that she was like his two previous wives, who had both cheated on him.

Finally, researchers subject their work to peer review. This helps researchers identify biases, illogical reasoning, or mistaken assumptions in each other's work. In our daily lives, we are not always willing to have others critically examine our thinking. Therefore, our biases, illogical reasoning, or poor assumptions may go unchallenged. In clinical work, seeking consultation with peers or supervisors can be a way of seeking peer review.

If we keep these principles in mind, we will be less likely to make errors in our own everyday pursuit of knowledge both inside and outside the therapy office. As you learn more about research concepts, we will help you see their relevance to the therapy process. Indeed, one of the goals of this book is to sharpen your critical thinking skills as a therapist by showing you how researchers try to gain knowledge.

FALSE DICHOTOMIES AND FALSE BELIEFS

If research is so valuable, then why are therapists so reluctant to learn research? One reason is that many clinicians have misconceptions about research. In this section we will explore and challenge some of these misconceptions.

Many therapists have been socialized to see research and clinical work as separate domains. It is not uncommon for undergraduate psychology students to observe that their faculty fall into two distinct camps—those that do research and those that do clinical work. This only reinforces the belief that research and clinical practice are independent of each other.

This belief has the unfortunate consequence of erecting a barrier between the two worlds. As a result, some clinicians question how much research can inform clinical work (Dattilio, Piercy, & Davis, 2014; Williams et al., 2006). They may believe, for example, that therapy is more of an art than a science. However, we believe this is a false dichotomy. We do not believe using research means the clinician will simply become a technician who lifelessly applies manualized treatments to clients. Rather, we see practicing therapy as both an art and a science, and that science can inform the art of therapy. Being a master musician requires both technical skill and artistic ability. In a similar manner, we believe therapists can use research knowledge in combination with their clinical experience to maximize their effectiveness.

Many also assume researchers and clinicians think in different ways. However, there is considerable overlap between the critical thinking skills used by researchers and therapists. Researchers and clinicians may use different language to describe these skills, but they are similar if you look beneath the labels. For example, researchers use the term *internal validity* to describe accurately attributing cause and effect to a phenomenon. This is really no different from what therapists do during assessment when they try to identify the underlying causes to their clients' problems.

Another false belief regarding research is that it is a highly mathematical discipline. Many clinicians equate research with statistics. While it is true that many studies use statistics to analyze the results, research actually relies more on logic than math for its rigor. A cornerstone of research is establishing cause and effect through internal validity, which is determined through research design rather than mathematics. Although an advanced understanding of research requires some mathematical knowledge, learning the fundamentals of research requires more of a conceptual than mathematical understanding.

Because many students equate research with statistics, many fear they will not have the necessary math skills to be successful in research. Their distaste for math does not improve their motivation to learn research. We want to assure you that we will discuss research and statistics from primarily a conceptual or logical standpoint, with very little reliance on mathematics.

PURPOSE AND PHILOSOPHY OF THIS BOOK

We anticipate that this book will be unlike other research methods texts you have read. The most obvious difference is that the book combines a discussion of both research methods and evidence-based practice. We believe combining these two elements will provide you with the best blueprint for applying research to your clinical work.

The first half of the book is devoted to teaching the fundamentals of research. In teaching research to our students, we often found that they came into our program with different levels of expertise or exposure to research. Our book will provide you with the essentials you need to effectively evaluate and apply research. Chapters 2–7 examine various research designs (e.g., experiments, surveys, qualitative research) that you will frequently encounter, while Chapter 8 examines values and ethical considerations in research. Chapters 9–11 provide a user-friendly introduction into descriptive and inferential statistics.

You will notice that the chapters in the first half of the book follow a set structure. Each chapter begins with a brief introduction and overview of the key concepts in the chapter. For those who have a strong background in research, the overview may be a sufficient refresher before exploring the application section. For those who are less familiar with the topic, the overview can orient you to the major ideas you will be learning. The overview is followed by the "Basics" section, which goes into more depth in discussing the key chapter concepts. This section is not intended to give you enough technical details to do research or statistical analyses, but it will provide you the necessary knowledge you need to understand research studies when you read them. The chapter concludes with an "Application" section. In this section, you will learn how to evaluate a study based on the chapter's concepts. It also explores how the concepts can be applied to your clinical work.

The second half of the book focuses on evidence-based practice (EBP), which will explore in detail a process for integrating research into your therapy. The first EBP chapter (12) will provide an overview of EBP and introduce you to the five A's (Ask, Acquire, Appraise, Apply, and Analyze and adjust). Subsequent chapters (13–18) will explore the A's in more detail. The book concludes with a chapter (19) on contextual factors that influence EBP, and how these factors may impact EBP in the future as it continues to evolve.

Our goal throughout the book is to present the concepts in a simple and straightforward manner. We are attempting to make the ideas as accessible as possible. You will notice, for example, that we often use metaphors and examples from everyday life to help you connect with the ideas. We also use numerous vignettes throughout the book to illustrate how research principles can be applied clinically. The use of vignettes is consistent with our philosophy that this is as much a clinical book as it is a research book. You will discover that many of the concepts and critical thinking skills that researchers use can be beneficial to clinicians. As you read the book, you may come to appreciate that the divide between research and clinical practice is not as great as you once thought.

At the end of the book you will find appendices we believe will be valuable references to you. The first appendix summarizes the key ideas from the EBP portion of the book, in essence a "pocket guide" for EBP. The second appendix list questions you may want to consider when evaluating research. The last appendix contains further resources on EBP you may want to explore. Key terms or concepts in the book that are highlighted in bold are found in the glossary, along with brief definitions.

ASSUMPTIONS

Several assumptions inform how we have written the book. First, we believe applying research to clinical work presents many complexities and challenges, which we will discuss throughout the book. We attempt to provide practical guidance on how to navigate these challenges. In spite of these challenges, we believe the effort invested in applying research to clinical work is worth it.

In addition, we recognize that most therapists have limited time and resources (Sandberg, Johnson, Robila, & Miller, 2002). As a busy clinician, you may find it difficult to set aside time to implement EBP. We try to show respect for your time by offering clear and concise guidelines for applying research. We also offer possible strategies that you can use to be most efficient in accessing and applying research.

We also recognize that not all research is of high quality. When using research, we believe in the old adage "Buyer beware!" Research is like the Internet in many ways. The Internet has made valuable knowledge more easily available to individuals. Through information on the Internet, one of us was able to diagnose why his dishwasher was not properly working. Furthermore, he was able to repair it with the guidance of a YouTube video. Yet, we also know that we have to be careful of the information on the Internet because it may be inaccurate or misleading. Research literature is much the same. Therefore, we will equip you with the knowledge and skills you need to critically evaluate research.

There is also debate in the field about what kind of research can be used in EBP. Some believe only findings from randomized experiments or clinical trials should be used in EBP. We agree that this type of research is the gold standard when evaluating treatments. However, we also believe this is a rather narrow definition of how research can inform clinical work (Dattilio et al., 2014). Other types of research can offer helpful insights regarding assessment, family dynamics, factors associated with mental illness, and the therapy process (just to name a few examples). Therefore, our position is that a variety of quantitative and qualitative research designs can provide valuable information depending upon the questions we are asking.

Earlier we noted that research is one of many potential sources of knowledge that can inform our clinical knowledge. Research should not necessarily replace these other sources of knowledge. Rather, we believe research findings can and should be integrated with other sources of information (e.g., clinical experience, intuition, knowledge of the client) to guide our clinical decision making.

Finally, you may notice that we make frequent reference throughout the book to EBP in the medical field. The primary reason is that the medical field is on the forefront of integrating EBP into clinical care. The medical field is often more advanced in developing EBP tools and guides than the mental health field. Therefore, we believe mental health professionals can benefit from being familiar with these tools. Furthermore, medical databases may have valuable research for mental health professionals, particularly in treating psychiatric illnesses. Yet, we also recognize that there are important differences between the medical and mental health professions that must be acknowledged. For example, the medical literature is more likely to focus on medications rather than psychotherapy for treating psychiatric illness. We have attempted to take the best in EBP practice in medicine while remaining true to what is unique to psychotherapy.

CONCLUSION

Learning research is a lot like having a cross-cultural experience as a traveler. When we visit a foreign land, initially the customs and language may seem strange and difficult to understand. Chapters 2–11 will introduce you to the customs and practices of research. Although the language and terms may seem foreign at first, we will help translate them so you can comprehend them. Once you get through the language barrier, you will discover many commonalities between how researchers and clinicians relate to the world.

Traveling to another culture can be an enriching experience. You can come away with a better understanding of your own culture by comparing it to the new culture you visited. It is our hope that you will have a similar experience as you learn more about research. Chapters 12–19 on EBP will help you build a bridge between research and your clinical world. So, let us begin the journey.

PART I

Research Foundations

CHAPTER 2

Measurement

Robert comes into therapy one day and reports to you that he is feeling down. What goes through your mind as he shares this with you? Perhaps you ask yourself, "What does he mean by this? Is he simply telling me he is having a bad day, or is he telling me he is depressed?" If he thinks he is depressed, you will likely ask him what his symptoms are. You may even consider giving him an instrument that assesses for depression. This can help you confirm whether Robert is depressed and its severity.

Both therapists and researchers are interested in measuring psychological phenomena like depression. We attach labels to represent these complex phenomena, which researchers call *constructs*. To measure constructs, we look for indicators that are associated with the phenomenon. These indicators can be used to create instruments that measure constructs. In the case of depression, we can look for psychological or behavioral signs such as sad affect, anhedonia, problems with sleep, or eating disturbances.

Developing these instruments requires a number of considerations. First, we must clearly define the construct. What constitutes depression, and how is it different from other disorders? Next, we must determine the best way to measure our construct. This will require attention to a number of factors. For example, will we want to assess the individual's thoughts, emotions, or behaviors? Is a single question adequate, or do we need to ask multiple questions to accurately capture what is going on? Will our question(s) be sensitive enough to distinguish individuals with various degrees of depression?

15

In this chapter, we will explore the importance of assessing the reliability, validity, and dimensions of multi-item scales. Different types of reliability look at various aspects of consistency. For reliability, we want to know if all the items in the instrument measure the same construct (internal reliability), if the instrument yields a consistent result over time (test–retest reliability), and in the case of behavior coding systems, we want to know if different raters code what is observed in the same manner (interrater reliability). We assess validity to ensure the instrument is measuring what we intended it to measure. Some forms of establishing validity are based on judgment (face, content), and others are based on empirical testing (criterion, construct). Finally, statistical techniques such as factor analysis or principal components analysis allow us to look at what items most closely correlate[1] with one another to determine whether one or more dimensions exist.

THE BASICS OF MEASUREMENT

There are three basics steps researchers go through when developing an instrument to measure a construct: (1) defining the construct, (2) creating the instrument, and (3) evaluating the new instrument.

Defining Constructs

Constructs are labels used to represent a phenomenon. Constructs are abstract concepts rather than physical properties (e.g., weight, length, chemical composition) that can be directly measured. Love, intelligence, and marital satisfaction are examples of constructs. In the social sciences, we are primarily interested in measuring constructs.

Constructs can be defined in multiple ways. For example, how would you define love? Your definition of love may differ from another person's definition. Likewise, researchers may define constructs in different ways

---

[1] If this is your first introduction to research methods, you may be unfamiliar with the term *correlate*, which means changes in one variable are associated with changes in another variable. The strength of the association or relationship is reflected by the correlation coefficient, which can range from 0 to 1 (with higher numbers indicating a stronger relationship) and can be either positive or negative. A positive correlation means that increasing scores on one variable are associated with increasing scores on a second variable (e.g., quality of communication and marital satisfaction). A negative correlation means that increasing scores on one variable are associated with decreasing scores on the other variable (level of violence and marital satisfaction). We will discuss correlations in more detail in Chapter 10.

based on their theoretical orientation. The complex nature of many constructs can also make them difficult to define. Love is a broad concept that can encompass feelings between romantic partners, a parent and a child, and friends. When defining a construct, you may need to articulate how it is distinct from other related constructs. For example, how is love different from infatuation?

Creating Instruments

Once the construct has been defined, the researcher then decides on a strategy for measuring it. This involves a number of considerations, which are often interrelated.

Operationalizing the Construct

Researchers must choose which indicators they will use to measure or **operationalize** the construct. In other words, what thoughts, feelings, or behaviors can be used to reflect the construct? How the construct is operationalized may depend on how it is defined. For example, if marital satisfaction is defined as the extent to which an individual's expectations are met, then the instrument will focus on measuring perceptions rather than behaviors.

Method of Measurement

How the construct is operationalized will impact the researcher's method of measurement. If the construct is operationalized using private thoughts or emotions, then the researcher will typically rely on a self-report instrument. **Self-report instruments** ask individuals to volunteer what they are thinking, feeling, or doing. If the construct is operationalized using behaviors, then the researcher could either have individuals provide a self-report or directly observe their behaviors. When observing behaviors directly, researchers will often record into categories what they see using a **coding system** (see Chapter 7). For example, a researcher might record what behaviors the parent uses when interacting with a child, such as asking questions, offering praise, doing problem solving, or criticizing the child. Measuring physiological indicators (e.g., heart rate, stress hormones) is another potential method of measurement occasionally used in psychological or social science research. For example, Minuchin and his team used free fatty acids concentrations obtained through blood samples in one study to measure the level of emotional arousal that each family member was experiencing (Minuchin, 1974). By measuring the rise and fall in free fatty acids over time, they were able to measure the impact that conflict had on different family members.

Most constructs in our field are measured using self-report instruments because we are often interested in directly accessing the thoughts and emotions individuals are experiencing. Private behaviors like sexual activity are also generally measured using self-report methods. Furthermore, using observational measures can require a lot of effort because coders must be trained and coding behaviors can be time-consuming.

Minimizing Reactivity

Sometimes the act of measuring something changes it. Individuals who know they are being observed, for example, may not behave as they normally would. This effect is called **reactivity**, perhaps because people often react to the process of being assessed or measured. Researchers want to minimize reactivity to get a more accurate picture of how people really are.

Social desirability is the most common form of reactivity, and refers to individuals answering questions or behaving in a manner that makes them appear good. Social desirability leads individuals to overreport positive behaviors (e.g., charitable giving, voting) and to underreport negative behaviors (e.g., substance use, child abuse) so they can be viewed in a favorable manner.

Researchers use a variety of approaches to manage social desirability. Researchers will sometimes use observational measures because behavior is generally under less conscious control than what people report verbally. That is why if a person's body language appears to contradict what is being said, we are more likely to trust the nonverbal message. The risk, however, is that the inferences we draw from behaviors may not be as accurate as asking individuals directly what they are thinking or feeling. For self-report measures, the wording of questions can impact social desirability. In Chapter 4, we will discuss ways researchers can construct questions to minimize social desirability. Offering confidentiality or anonymity can also encourage individuals to be more honest. Some instruments include scales that allow one to measure the extent an individual is answering in a socially desirable way. For example, the Minnesota Multiphasic Personality Inventory (a measure of personality and psychopathology) includes scales that detect if individuals are underreporting psychological symptoms.

In addition to social desirability, demand characteristics and learning are two other forms of reactivity. **Demand characteristics** can occur when individuals provide answers they believe the researcher desires, perhaps to please the researcher or to avoid being judged. For example, respondents may report feeling better because they do not want to disappoint the researcher that they are still depressed despite receiving treatment. **Learning** results when the respondent gains knowledge or skills through being measured. This is most likely to occur if an instrument is administered more than once, resulting in improved performance on subsequent administrations through learning new information or repetitive practice.

Enhancing Sensitivity

Researchers want to be able to detect differences between individuals when measuring a construct, which is called **sensitivity**. A question that simply asks if an individual is happily or unhappily married would not be very sensitive because it would not differentiate between those who are extremely happy in their marriage from those who are moderately or mildly happy. Likewise, it would not distinguish between those who are somewhat unhappy and those who are highly distressed. The number of response choices can impact sensitivity. For example, sensitivity could be improved by adding more choices (e.g., extremely happy, very happy, somewhat happy, mixed, somewhat unhappy, very unhappy, extremely unhappy).

A single question is also less sensitive than a multi-item scale because there is a smaller range of scores. For a multi-item scale, the scores across a number of questions can be combined to provide a larger range of scores, thereby creating more degrees of difference. The Dyadic Adjustment Scale (Spanier, 1976), which can range from a score of 0 to a score of 151, would be a more sensitive measure of marital quality compared to our 7-point scale above.

However, multi-item scales can experience problems with sensitivity due to ceiling effects or floor effects. **Ceiling effects** arise when scores cluster on the high end of the scale. For example, if you think of a multiple-choice exam as a multi-item scale measuring student knowledge in a particular subject, then ceiling effects can arise if the exam is too easy and nearly everyone aces the exam. Hence, the exam would not distinguish between those who had mastered the material and those with a superficial knowledge of it. Conversely, **floor effects** would exist if scores clustered on the low end of the scale, which could arise if the exam is so difficult that everyone fails it. Inspecting the distribution of scores can detect if ceiling or floor effects exist.

Single-Item or Multi-Item Measure

When using a self-report measure, you must decide whether to use a single item or multiple items. Using a single item is the simplest approach, but it typically restricts one to measuring the construct in a global fashion (e.g., *How satisfied overall are you with your relationship?*). In contrast, multi-item scales allow you to measure the construct in more detail, which is helpful if the construct is complex and has multiple dimensions. For example, the McMaster Family Assessment Device (FAD) is a popular measure of family functioning (Epstein, Baldwin, & Bishop, 1983). The FAD has various subscales that allow one to assess different dimensions of family functioning, including problem solving, communication, roles, affective responsiveness, affective involvement, and behavior control. As discussed above, multi-item scales are often more sensitive than using a single question.

Because multi-item scales can add significantly to the length of a survey, researchers must be judicious in their use, and typically reserve them for the most important variables. Surveys may include a small number of multi-item scales, but primarily rely on single items to measure constructs to avoid making the survey too long.

Level of Measurement

When developing an instrument, the researcher must also decide what the level of measurement will be. This has implications for how sensitive a measure is, as well as the type of statistical analysis that is appropriate to use (which we discuss in more detail in Chapters 10 and 11).

The four levels of measurement are nominal, ordinal, interval, and ratio. The lowest level of measurement is **nominal**. Nominal variables do not have any numeric or quantitative properties, but simply assign names to the possible choices. Examples of nominal variables include marital status, gender, or religious affiliation.

The next level of measurement is **ordinal**, which is quantitative in nature and allows one to assign a rank order to values. Sports polls that rank the top teams are ordinal. An ordinal scale commonly used in research is the Likert scale, which asks individuals whether they strongly agree, agree, disagree, or strongly disagree with a statement. Most questions that offer responses stated in words rather than numeric scales (1–10) are ordinal, even if they suggest a possible frequency (e.g., frequently, often, seldom, never). The potential difficulty with ordinal variables is that the distance between the values is not known or it may be unequal. Using our sports poll example, the top two teams may be close in performance, but a big gap may exist between the second and third ranked teams. This problem is addressed in the next level of measurement.

In an **interval** level of measurement, the distance (interval) between values is equal. Temperature using Fahrenheit or Celsius is an interval scale. The distance between 36 and 37 degrees is the same as the distance between other values, such as 86 and 87 degrees. However, the designation of zero is arbitrary in interval scales. Zero in our thermometer example does not represent the absence of heat. As a result, you cannot say that 60 degrees is twice as warm as 30 degrees. In a similar manner, you cannot say that someone with an IQ score of 150 is twice as smart as someone with a score of 75 because zero is arbitrary, and it does not correspond with an individual having no intelligence.

Although most multi-item scales are composed of items that strictly speaking are ordinal in nature (e.g., Likert questions), the total score can often be treated like an interval level of measurement. That is because the total scores begin to approximate an interval scale as you sum the scores across a number of items in a scale. This is important because it allows researchers to use more sophisticated statistical analyses that require an interval level of measurement.

The highest level of measurement is **ratio**, and it possesses both equal intervals and an absolute zero. Variables such as income, age, or height are ratio because zero has real meaning (e.g., the complete absence of a property) rather than being arbitrarily assigned. Because ratio variables have an absolute value, it is possible to make meaningful comparisons. For example, we can state that an individual has twice the income of another. Table 2.1 summarizes the properties that each level of measurement possesses.

Evaluating Scales

As discussed above, sensitivity and reactivity are two important characteristics to consider when developing an instrument. In addition, researchers typically evaluate two other properties of multi-item scales: reliability and validity. A researcher may also determine if a scale has

TABLE 2.1. Properties of Different Levels of Measurement

Level of measurement	Does it possess this property?	
Nominal	Rank order?	No
	Equal interval?	No
	Absolute zero?	No
Ordinal	Rank order?	Yes
	Equal interval?	No
	Absolute zero?	No
Interval	Rank order?	Yes
	Equal interval?	Yes
	Absolute zero?	No
Ratio	Rank order?	Yes
	Equal interval?	Yes
	Absolute zero?	Yes

multiple dimensions, and which items are most closely associated with each dimension.

Reliability

Reliability refers to whether the instrument gives a consistent answer. Table 2.2 summarizes the three types of reliability. One type of reliability is **internal reliability**, which assesses if all the items are consistent in measuring the same construct. For example, if you are developing an instrument to measure depression, then all of the items should relate to symptoms of depression. You would not want to include items that relate to other disorders, which would negatively impact its internal consistency.

Internal reliability can be assessed using different methods. The most frequently used method is the Cronbach's alpha, which is based on how strongly items correlate with one another. Items that strongly correlate with one another will yield higher values, indicating greater internal reliability. A variation of the Cronbach's alpha, called the Küder–Richardson, is used if the items are dichotomous (e.g., true/false, yes/no). Another method, called the split-half, is sometimes reported, and simply looks at how strongly two halves of the instrument (e.g., odd vs. even items) correlate with one another. Scores from both halves should

TABLE 2.2. Different Types of Reliability

Internal reliability: Are the items in an instrument consistent in measuring the same construct? The three ways to measure internal reliability are Cronbach's alpha, split-half, and Küder–Richardson (for dichotomous items).

Test–retest reliability: Does the instrument yield consistent scores over time?

Interrater reliability: Are raters consistent in how they categorize behaviors using a coding system?

---

strongly correlate with one another if they are measuring the same construct. In all three methods, scores vary between zero and one, with higher values representing greater internal consistency. Reliability scores of .80 and above are considered good for research purposes, while scores of .90 and above are usually expected for instruments used for clinical application.

Another form of reliability is **test–retest reliability**, which measures the consistency of scores over time. Researchers evaluate test–retest reliability by giving the instrument to the same set of individuals at two different times (e.g., 2 or 4 weeks apart). For many constructs like IQ, you would not anticipate a significant change of scores over time. Therefore, there should be a strong correlation between scores at both points in time if the instrument has good test–retest reliability. Ideally test–retest correlations will be .80 and above, with scores ranging from zero to one.

For observational measures, **interrater reliability** evaluates if there is consistency across raters in how they code or categorize behaviors. For example, if two coders are observing a parent–child interaction, they ideally will be consistent in recording when the parent made a critical comment about the child if that is a category in the coding scheme. Ideally interrater reliabilities will be .80 or above across all categories, although the reliabilities for specific behaviors or categories may be lower.

Validity

In addition to evaluating the reliability of an instrument, the researcher must also evaluate its **validity** (sometimes called measurement validity to distinguish it from internal validity and external validity). For an instrument to be valid, it must be measuring the intended construct. An instrument for measuring depression would be invalid if it were actually assessing anxiety rather than depression.

To be valid, an instrument must also be reliable. A depression scale that gives you widely different scores every time you take it will not give valid results. However, an instrument can be reliable and not valid. A reliable instrument may consistently give the wrong answer if it is not measuring the proper construct.

There are multiple ways to demonstrate an instrument is valid. **Face validity** simply requires that one look at the instrument items to judge if it appears to be valid. This is the least rigorous form of validity. **Content validity** evaluates if the instrument includes all the important aspects of the construct. For example, a depression scale should include all the important symptoms of depression and not overlook any important ones. In another example, Spanier (1976) felt previous research had overlooked the importance of commitment when measuring marital adjustment. Therefore, when he developed the Dyadic Adjustment Scale, he added commitment to enhance the content validity of the scale. Content validity is established by having experts review the instrument to ensure it includes the necessary concepts (or excludes items that do not apply).

While face and content validity are based on judgment, criterion and construct validity use an empirical approach to establish validity. **Criterion validity** is demonstrated by showing the new instrument relates to another criterion or indicator in an anticipated manner. For example, you could demonstrate the SAT is a valid measure of college preparedness by showing that SAT scores accurately predict students' later college GPAs. When the criterion variable is measured in the future (e.g., college GPA), then this is an example of **predictive validity**, which is a subtype of criterion validity.

Concurrent validity is another subtype of criterion validity, and is established by correlating the new instrument with a criterion variable known concurrently or at the same time (rather than the future). One way to demonstrate concurrent validity is to confirm that two groups you logically expect to be different do indeed score differently on the instrument. Establishing criterion validity in this manner is sometimes called *known-groups validity*. For example, Spanier (1976) showed the Dyadic Adjustment Scale scores were significantly different for married and divorced individuals. Concurrent validity can also be demonstrated by correlating the new instrument with an established way of measuring the same construct. If you administer a new depression inventory and the Beck Depression Inventory together, then a strong correlation between the two would provide evidence for concurrent validity.

Construct validity is the second approach to establishing validity empirically, which is accomplished by showing that the instrument relates to other constructs as theoretically expected. If an instrument for measuring depression has construct validity, then you would expect higher scores for depression to be associated with lower life satisfaction scores. Conversely, you would not expect your measure of depression to correlate with other constructs where no relationship is anticipated based on theory.

Another way to establish construct validity is to show that the instrument strongly correlates with another way of measuring the same construct, which is often referred to as **convergent validity**.[2] For example, Spanier (1976) showed the Dyadic Adjustment Scale scores strongly correlated with the Marital Adjustment Test, the previous gold standard for measuring marital adjustment. In contrast, **discriminant validity** (sometimes called *divergent validity*) confirms that the instrument does not strongly correlate with instruments that measure other constructs. Discriminant validity is often used in combination with convergent validity. The idea is that the instrument should strongly correlate with alternative ways of measuring the same construct (convergent validity), but have a weaker correlation with instruments that measure different constructs (discriminant validity). One would anticipate that a new scale for depression would strongly correlate with other measures of depression, but have a weaker correlation with measures for anxiety or self-esteem.

Factorial validity is a third potential way to establish construct validity. This is demonstrated by running a **factor analysis** (described in more detail below) to confirm the instrument behaves theoretically as expected with regards to its internal structure or dimensions. Spanier (1976) argued for the factorial validity of the Dyadic Adjustment Scale because factor analysis verified the existence of three factors (dyadic satisfaction, dyadic cohesion, and dyadic consensus) that were theoretically predicted.[3] If an instrument has factorial validity, items that are predicted to relate to a particular dimension should have a stronger correlation with one another than with items related to other dimensions.

Table 2.3 summarizes the different approaches to establishing validity for a measure. Do not be surprised if researchers sometimes refer to the various ways of establishing criterion and construct validity using

---

[2] As discussed earlier, some researchers view this as a way of establishing concurrent validity.

[3] A new factor, affectional expression, was also uncovered through the factor analysis.

TABLE 2.3. Methods for Establishing the Validity of an Instrument

Approach to establishing validity	Name
Based on one's judgment, does the instrument appear to be a valid measure?	Face validity
Based on expert review, does the instrument cover all of the relevant domains of the construct?	Content validity
Does the instrument relate to some criterion in the expected manner?	Criterion validity
Does the instrument relate to some criterion measured *in the future* in the expected manner?	Predictive validity
Does the instrument relate to some criterion measured *at the same time* in the expected manner?	Concurrent validity
Does the instrument relate to other constructs in the manner that one would expect?	Construct validity
Does the instrument strongly correlate with other measures of the *same* construct?	Convergent validity
Does the instrument *not* strongly correlate with measures of different constructs?	Discriminant, divergent validity
Does factor analysis reveal the internal structure to be consistent with what is theoretically expected?	Factorial validity

different labels, although an attempt has been made to use the most common conventions here. There also can be a difference of opinion on whether one way of establishing validity is a form of criterion or construct validity. For example, some view correlating a new instrument with an established measure as a form of criterion validity (concurrent), while others view it as a form of construct validity (convergent). Regardless of the labels attached, the important thing to understand is the underlying logic behind the researcher's attempt to establish validity.

Dimensionality of the Scale

One advantage of multi-item scales is that they may permit you to look at different aspects or dimensions of a construct, thus allowing a more sophisticated understanding of a phenomenon. The Dyadic Adjustment Scale (Spanier, 1976) has four subscales that correspond with four dimensions: (1) satisfaction with the relationship (dyadic satisfaction), (2) the extent to which the couple agrees on important issues in the relationship (dyadic consensus), (3) how much the couple engages in activities together (dyadic cohesion), and (4) the quality of their physical/sexual relationship (affectional expression). Using factor analysis (or principal components analysis[4]), researchers can assess if a scale has multiple dimensions. Factor analysis can be used in an exploratory manner to uncover possible dimensions, or it can be used to establish factorial validity by confirming the internal structure is consistent with what the researcher predicted.

Table 2.4 shows the results from a principal components analysis where the researchers developed items to measure individuals' motivations for cohabitating (Murrow & Shi, 2010). The analysis uncovered that the items clustered around three factors. The results also show how strongly each item correlates with each factor. These correlations are called *factor loadings*, with values that range from 0 to 1 and can be either positive or negative. Ideally, each item will heavily correlate with only one factor, and have a weak correlation with other factors (although this is not always the case). For example, items 1 through 3 strongly correlate with factor 1, but weakly correlate with the other two factors. To make it easier to see which items primarily load on each factor, factor loadings above .40 may be highlighted.[5] Alternatively, factor loadings less than .40 may be left blank.

As a final step, the researcher will determine if there is a common theme to the items that load on a factor, and then label the factor accordingly. In this example, items 1–3 cluster together on a factor because they all relate to cohabitation being a precursor to getting married. Inspection of items 4–7 reveals a common theme of viewing cohabitation as a trial marriage, and items 8 and 9 relate to the convenience of cohabitating while dating.

Factor analysis and principal components analysis can be used to identify items that do not strongly correlate with other items, and thus may not belong in the scale. For example, in Table 2.4 it is evident the last item does not strongly load on any of the three factors. As a result, the researchers eliminated this item. An item that does not strongly correlate with other items is only weakly measuring the construct or is measuring a different construct. Thus, eliminating the item will improve the internal reliability of the scale.

---

[4]Although there are some differences, both factor analysis and principal components analysis share many similarities and can be used for similar purposes.

[5]Sometimes loadings of .30 rather than .40 may be used as the cutoff.

TABLE 2.4. Assessing Dimensions of a Scale for Measuring Purpose of Cohabitation

	Factor Loadings		
Item	Factor 1: Precursor to Marriage	Factor 2: Trial Marriage	Factor 3: Coresidential Dating
1. I want to live with my partner instead of getting married.*	−.896	−.233	.029
2. Living together is a better choice for me than being married.*	−.875	−.007	.072
3. I am living with my partner because we are engaged or planning to get married.	.678	.192	.031
4. Living together will help me to know my partner better.	.048	.832	−.016
5. I want to test out living together before I make a further commitment to my partner.	.021	.818	.011
6. Living together is a trial run for marriage.	.206	.779	.039
7. If we are successful at living together, I think we will be successful at marriage.	.543	.618	.221
8. It is more convenient to live together than to live apart.	.043	−.012	.825
9. Living together made sense because of financial or economic reasons.	−.060	.025	.776
10. Living together shows my commitment to my partner.	.376	−.236	−.318

Note. Adapted from Murrow and Shi (2010). Reprinted with permission from Taylor & Francis. *www.informaworld.com.*

*Indicates item is reversed scored.

APPLICATION

Evaluating Measurement Issues in Research

There are a number of things you should consider when evaluating measurement issues for a study. For studies using existing measures, do you agree with how the researcher chose to measure key variables? For example, did the researcher's use of self-report and/or observational measures make sense? Likewise, did the researcher make appropriate use of single-item versus multi-item scales? If the researcher is analyzing data collected by someone else, the measures used may not be a perfect fit with the researcher's aims, which is often a limitation of analyzing secondary data.

If a new instrument was developed, did the researcher provide a clear rationale for why it needed to be created (e.g., measuring a new construct, addresses limitations of instruments for a similar construct)? Did the researcher clearly define the construct? Does the approach for operationalizing or measuring the construct make sense?

For new and existing multi-item scales, does the researcher provide evidence for their reliability? Internal reliabilities should be .80 and above. If test–retest reliability is reported, it should be .80 and above. For observational measures or coding systems, interrater reliabilities should generally be .80 and above, although some behaviors or categories may be lower.

The researcher should also provide evidence for the validity of multi-item scales. The more forms of validity that are evaluated, the greater confidence one can have in the instrument. For existing instruments, the researcher may simply reference previous studies that assessed the reliability and validity of the instrument rather than describe the properties in the report.

Are there any potential concerns with sensitivity or reactivity? As discussed earlier, issues of sensitivity are more likely to arise when measuring constructs using a single item. Reactivity in the form of social desirability is most likely to arise when measuring sensitive topics. Has the researcher taken steps to minimize social desirability (e.g., wording of questions, offers confidentiality or anonymity)? Also, is there the potential for demand characteristics or learning to impact the findings?

Evaluating Assessment Instruments

The above discussion relates to instruments used in a research study. These same ideas apply when evaluating assessment instruments used in clinical practice. In fact, many instruments initially developed for research purposes can have clinical utility. It is important that assessment instruments have good reliability and validity. Higher standards are needed for assessment instruments that are used to make decisions that impact individuals' lives. Therefore, internal reliabilities of at least .90 are considered necessary for instruments used clinically, rather than the .80 required for research purposes.

The Therapist as the Assessment Instrument

Many of the concepts we discussed in regards to measurement in research can also be applied when we are asking clients assessment questions. When we ask clients about their experiences, we need to be aware they may define key words (constructs) differently from us. Consider a simple question like "How often do you and your partner fight?" Is any disagreement considered a fight, or is it a fight only if the disagreement escalates to individuals being angry or yelling at each other?

Measurement concepts can inform how therapists ask questions or conduct assessments. Content validity encourages us to consider if we are considering all the relevant aspects of a phenomenon. When assessing depression, for example, do we focus primarily on the mood symptoms associated with depression and exclude assessment of physical symptoms? When we ask questions, are we asking them in such a way to maximize sensitivity? For example, Roxanne could ask her clients if they are committed to the relationship, in which the clients are likely to answer yes or no. It is better to ask clients to rate on a scale of 1 to 10 their level of commitment. This will be more sensitive to different levels of commitment, and it will more accurately reflect the varying levels of ambivalence of many individuals who seek couple therapy.

Therapists must always be mindful of reactivity during assessment, especially social desirability. Clients may not always be completely honest in answering your questions to maintain a positive image. How we ask questions may help reduce social desirability. In addition, establishing a strong and nonjudgmental therapeutic relationship is essential to minimizing social desirability. Demand characteristics can also occur. For example, clients may report things are getting better so as not to disappoint their therapist. Sometimes simply asking a question introduces a new angle or perspective to a client, which creates learning. However, learning is less of a problem in the clinical arena, and is often a desirable outcome. Keeping these measurement concepts in mind can help you be more effective as a therapist, particularly during assessment.

CHAPTER 3

Internal Validity and Experiments

You are watching your TV, when suddenly the picture goes black. You immediately begin to wonder what happened. Did your TV just die? Is it a problem with the satellite or cable feed? Or, maybe it is a problem with the station you are watching. You get up to change the channel to see if the problem is happening on other channels. To your relief, the other channels appear to be working. Therefore, you conclude the station you are watching is experiencing technical difficulties.

This everyday example illustrates the principle of internal validity, which is concerned with identifying the underlying causes of a phenomenon. When there are competing explanations for why something has occurred, running experiments can help us identify the underlying cause. In our TV example, we ran an experiment by changing only the channel, keeping other variables the same (the TV, the cable or satellite feed). Using this approach, we were able to conclude the station supplying the signal was the problem. Thus, experiments are invaluable in helping us establish internal validity.

However, running experiments in the social sciences is more complicated than simply changing the channel on a TV. This chapter will examine how researchers conduct experiments when studying human behavior or evaluating therapy treatments. The randomized controlled trial (RCT) is considered the gold standard for how to run experiments. The RCT includes two or more comparison groups (e.g., treatment vs. no treatment control) where only one variable is changed and all other variables are held constant. It also includes random assignment of the subjects to the different groups to ensure that the groups are equivalent except for the one variable being manipulated.

THE BASICS OF INTERNAL VALIDITY AND EXPERIMENTS

Internal Validity

Internal validity is concerned with accurately identifying cause and effect variables. Because human behavior is complicated, it may be difficult to determine cause and effect in relationships. There may be several competing explanations for why something happens. In therapy, it may be difficult to determine the underlying causes to our clients' problems, or which of our interventions actually helped to create change.

Obviously there must be some association or correlation between two variables that have a cause and effect relationship. However, internal validity may be difficult to establish between the two variables because the direction of the cause and effect may be unclear. Does A cause B, or does B cause A? For example, what explains the relationship between mental health problems and divorce (Amato, 2010)? Do individuals with mental health problems have a higher risk for divorce, or does the stress of divorce create a higher incidence of mental health problems?

A correlation between two variables does not guarantee a cause and effect relationship exists. There may be a **spurious relationship**, where the relationship between the two variables arises because both are caused by a third variable. Ice cream consumption and the sale of sunglasses may be correlated with one another. However, the sale of one does not cause the sale of the other. Rather, rising and falling seasonal temperatures drive the sales of both.

In the above example it may be easy to see a spurious relationship exists. However, the presence of a spurious relationship may not always be obvious. For example, a relationship between cohabitation and poorer marital outcomes such as distress and divorce has been documented. What accounts for this relationship? Does the experience of cohabiting increase individuals' risk for marital difficulties? Or, is it possible the relationship is spurious? A spurious relationship could arise if the attributes that make individuals more likely to cohabitate also make them more likely to have problems in marriage. For example, it is possible that individuals who have a weaker commitment to marriage (or their partner) are more likely to cohabitate, and are also more likely to experience divorce due to their weaker commitment. Current research suggests both scenarios may be true. Cohabitating may lead to poorer marital outcomes, particularly if the couple "slides" into marriage (Stanley, Rhoades, & Markman, 2006). However, there is also evidence that the individuals who cohabitate are different from those who do not, and that these differences may partially account for the poorer marital outcomes among those who have cohabitated.

Experiments help us address issues relating to internal validity in two ways. First, they control the sequence of events, which eliminates questions regarding the direction of causality. The researcher selects one variable to change first, and then observes if it had the anticipated effect on the second variable. Second, the researcher controls for other extraneous variables, eliminating the potential for spurious relationships.

Threats to Internal Validity

Imagine that you have developed a new treatment approach that helps individuals struggling to recover from divorce. You initially administer the Beck Depression Inventory (BDI) to 25 individuals as a pretest to measure their level of distress. You then have them participate in a 12-week program on divorce adjustment. After completing the program, you have the individuals retake the BDI again as a posttest to see if their depression has improved. You discover that the average BDI score has decreased by several points. Therefore, you conclude your program is a big success. Are you justified in concluding your program is a success?

Researchers would be hesitant to conclude that the program caused the reduction in depression scores based on the design you used. They would first want to rule out other explanations for the change. What might be other competing explanations, which researchers refer to as **threats to internal validity**?

It is possible that **history** may account for the change. History refers to external events that happen during an experiment that can influence the results. For example, if you began your study in November, individuals may be more depressed than usual due to the holidays. When you retest individuals 3 months later, their depression may have improved because the holidays have passed. Or, perhaps some individuals began new love relationships during treatment, which may have lifted their depression.

Maturation is another potential threat to internal validity. Maturation refers to the fact that people inevitably change over time. This is particularly true for children, who naturally mature and change. However, maturation can also apply to adults. The old adage "time heals all wounds" is an example of maturation. The passage of time rather than your program may have helped individuals in your study better adjust to being divorced.

You would also need to rule out **mortality** as a threat. Mortality occurs when individuals drop out of a study due to death or some other reason. In our example, individuals with severe depression may be especially prone to dropping out because a lack of motivation is a symptom of depression. If the most depressed individuals drop out of the study, then average depression scores could improve even if others showed no improvement.

Effects from **testing** due to reactivity (see Chapter 2) may be another threat to internal validity. Perhaps individuals are embarrassed that they are still struggling with the divorce despite being in an intervention program. Social desirability may lead individuals to underreport depressive symptoms in an attempt to look better than they are doing in reality. Or, demand characteristics may lead individuals to report doing better than they are in order to please you because they know the program is important to you. It is also possible that learning may have occurred through retesting. Perhaps individuals learned from taking the depression inventory that they are depressed, and then pursued other strategies for addressing depression on their own.

Instrument decay can be another potential threat related to measurement, which can occur if the way the outcome variable is measured changes over time. This is more likely to happen when using human observers. For example, if you used raters to code depressive behaviors rather than the BDI, it is possible that the skill of the raters might change over time. Burnout may lead raters to be less conscientious in noting depressive behaviors, leading to an artificial improvement in depression scores. Conversely, raters may become more skilled at noting depressive symptoms, making it appear that individuals had declined, when indeed there was no change or perhaps even improvement.

Finally, **statistical regression to the mean** has to be ruled out as a possible cause for the improvement. If individuals are selected to participate in a study based on their extreme scores, regression to the mean may occur upon retesting. Some scores are initially extreme due in part to chance factors. For example, some of the individuals may have depression scores below their normal baseline because they were having a particularly bad day. Upon retesting, they return to their normal baseline, making it appear that they had improved. A popular example of regression to the mean is the *Sports Illustrated* jinx (Cozby, 2004), where the performance of many athletes seems to decline after appearing on the cover of the magazine. These athletes are often chosen because they are experiencing a hot streak. However, they inevitably return to their baseline in performance, which many misattribute to the jinx.

One way to eliminate these threats is to include a comparison group. Often this is a no-treatment control group. However, an alternative treatment could be used as the comparison group, particularly if the goal is to demonstrate that a new treatment is better than the current best practice. If one of the above threats is the underlying cause for the change, then both groups should be equally impacted. Thus, you can rule out these factors as the reason for the change if you still find a difference between the treatment and comparison groups.

However, **selection bias** may be a possible threat to internal validity even when using a comparison group. A selection bias occurs when the individuals in the groups are different in some important way, such as symptom severity. It then becomes difficult to determine if the results are due to preexisting differences between the subjects or due to treatment effects. If a greater proportion of depressed individuals happen to be in the control group, then the treatment group may appear to be better simply because it had fewer depressed individuals. The risk for a selection bias is high if subjects have chosen the treatment they will receive. A researcher who compares the effectiveness of two premarital counseling programs may encounter a selection bias if comparing a 1-day workshop with a program where couples meet weekly over 8 weeks. This is because couples willing to invest in an 8-week period may be more highly motivated than couples choosing the 1-day program.

The way to avoid a selection bias is to randomly assign individuals to the various groups. This reduces the risk that groups will be significantly different. The larger the groups, the better randomization works to ensure the groups are equivalent.[1] The use of random assignment and a comparison group is considered an ideal experimental design (see further discussion below), and is referred to as a **randomized controlled trial** (RCT).

Sometimes it is not possible to randomly assign individuals to groups,

---

[1] With small groups, chance factors may make the groups nonequivalent. However, this probability becomes smaller as the size of the groups increases.

in which case a **quasi-experimental design** is the next best option. In this design, the groups receive both a pretest and posttest. By administering a pretest, the researcher can compare the groups to see if they are equivalent before the experiment begins. In the divorce therapy study, you could see if the average pretest depression scores are equivalent for both groups. It is possible, however, that the groups may be nonequivalent on an important variable not measured through pretesting. Perhaps the two groups are different on the average length of time since divorce. Those who have struggled with the divorce for a longer period of time may be more difficult to treat. Therefore, random assignment gives us the greatest confidence that the groups are equivalent.

Experimental Designs

As we described above, the two essential ingredients for an experimental design are a comparison group and random assignment. The experimental design may include pretesting, or it may not. Pretesting can be used to confirm the groups are equivalent, although this may not be necessary with the random assignment of a large pool of subjects. It also enables the researcher to measure the magnitude of change between pretest and posttest scores, and not just if the posttest scores are different between the groups. Pretesting also allows you to evaluate mortality effects to see if individuals who drop out of the study are different from those who remain.

Pretesting does carry some potential disadvantages. The most obvious is that it requires more effort and perhaps expense to do. Pretesting may also interact with the treatment, potentially heightening the effect of the treatment. Pretesting may sensitize or alert participants to what the researcher is studying, leading them to change their behavior. One way to evaluate if this is happening is to conduct a **Solomon four-group design**. Using this design, both the experimental and comparison groups are conducted with and without pretesting, creating four groups. The two experimental groups can be compared with one another to see if pretesting created a difference. The same can be done with the two comparison groups to see if pretesting changed the results.

Although randomized controlled experiments are powerful designs, they are not immune to experiencing other threats to internal validity. One possible threat is the **placebo effect**, which can result in the individuals improving simply because they expect to benefit from the treatment. It is the expectancy of change rather than the actual intervention itself that leads to improvement. This placebo effect must be considered when the comparison group is a no-treatment control. In pharmaceutical research, individuals in the no-treatment group may be given sugar pills to control for the placebo effect. Thus, both groups are equally likely to experience the placebo effect because both are receiving pills. Any difference between the treatment and no-treatment group can then be attributed to the actual medication effects. Unfortunately, it can be difficult to develop a proper placebo control when designing experiments to evaluate therapy interventions.

Randomized controlled experiments can suffer from other threats to internal validity. For example, if the therapists who deliver one treatment are more experienced than the therapists delivering an alternative treatment, then differences in effectiveness could arise due to this factor rather than differences in the treatments. Table 3.1 briefly summarizes other potential threats to internal validity that may be encountered in experimental designs.

Repeated-Measures or Within-Subjects Designs

Experiments can also be designed with subjects acting as their own comparison group. These are called **repeated-measures** or **within-subjects** designs. In these designs, subjects are exposed to more than one condition, and then differences in their responses are measured. For example, individuals may first be exposed to deep breathing to reduce stress. Subjects are then exposed to muscle relaxation to see how it compares to deep breathing in reducing stress.

This type of design has two key advantages. First, it tends to be more sensitive than the traditional experimental design. In the traditional experimental design, differences between groups can arise because the conditions are different, and also because the groups contain different individuals.[2] However, in a repeated-measures design, each person serves as his or her own control. As a result, any differences that are found can be attributed solely to the differences in conditions because variation from using different people in the groups has been eliminated. Second, a repeated-measures design requires fewer subjects, which can be an important factor if availability of subjects is limited. Twice as many subjects would be needed for a traditional experimental design that compares two conditions.

---

[2] The differences that arise from using different people in the groups will hopefully be small if the randomization of subjects works, especially if the groups are large enough.

TABLE 3.1. Potential Threats to Internal Validity for Randomized Controlled Experiments

Compensatory equalization. Providers of the treatment may attempt to offset a perceived inequality in treatments by offering those in the comparison group additional support or help. This can make it more difficult to find a difference between the treatment and comparison groups.[a]

Compensatory rivalry. This can occur when individuals in the comparison group attempt to offset a perceived inequality in treatment by working harder. Like compensatory equalization, this can make it more difficult to find a difference between the treatment and comparison groups.[a]

Demoralization. This is similar to compensatory rivalry, except individuals in the comparison group become demoralized, leading to poorer outcomes for them. This creates a bias in favor of finding a positive result for the treatment.[a]

Diffusion. This problem arises if some of the knowledge or interventions in the new treatment are also delivered to the comparison group. Diffusion can occur, for example, if therapists in a "treatment as usual" comparison group use some of the concepts or interventions used by the therapists in the new treatment group. Diffusion makes it difficult to uncover differences between the treatment and comparison groups.

Hawthorne effect. Individuals may change their behavior because they know they are being studied or observed. For example, individuals in the treatment group may improve because they are receiving attention. However, the control group does not improve because they are not receiving comparable attention, leading to a potential bias in favor of the treatment.

Selective mortality. This can arise if one group suffers from a higher attrition or mortality rate than the other, which can impact the findings. For example, if the most depressed individuals drop out of the treatment condition because they find it too difficult or strenuous, then this can inflate the posttest scores. Selective mortality can create a bias either for or against the treatment depending upon the nature of the selection effects on mortality for each group.

[a]In pharmaceutical research, double-blind studies are used to control for compensatory equalization, compensatory rivalry, and demoralization. In double-blind studies, neither the treatment providers nor the patients know who is receiving which treatment. Double-blind studies are difficult to implement in psychotherapy research.

A repeated-measures design is not feasible if the effects of the treatment are permanent or long lasting. For example, you cannot unlearn something. As a result, a repeated-measures design is less commonly used because most interventions are intended to create lasting change rather than produce temporary effects. Repeated-measures designs can also suffer from order effects, which result when subjects behave differently because of the order in which they received the conditions. For example, if a study measures performance on a task, individuals may do better on the second condition due to practice. Conversely, they may do worse after the second condition due to fatigue. Counterbalancing addresses this problem by having half the sample receive one condition first, while the other half receives the other condition first. Thus, order effects are equally likely to affect both conditions.

Strengths and Limitations of Experimental Research

As you read the chapters on other research designs, you will learn each design has strengths and limitations. One must match the type of design to the type of research question that needs to be answered. The key strength of experiments is their ability to rule out alternative explanations for cause and effect. In psychotherapy research, experiments are considered the gold standard for demonstrating that a treatment is effective, and that positive changes cannot be attributed to other factors. Therefore, experiments are considered the best design for establishing internal validity. However, it is not always feasible or ethical to test certain variables through experiments. Some variables such as temperament cannot be altered, making them difficult to study using experimental designs. Ethically it would be inappropriate to assign children to abusive and nonabusive parents to test the impact of physical abuse on child behavior. In these situations, researchers must rely on correlational research based on existing cases to study these phenomena.

Another potential criticism of experimental research is its artificiality. Researchers attempt to exert a great deal of control over all the variables in an attempt to isolate change in one variable. In real life, it is difficult to exert this level of control. This can be a concern when generalizing results from an experiment. Will a treatment only work in the laboratory under ideal conditions, or will the treatment effect be robust enough to be evident in real-life conditions?[3]

The above question has led to the distinction between two types of research—**efficacy** and **effectiveness research**. In efficacy research, treatments are evaluated in a highly controlled manner. For example, researchers can carefully monitor if the treatments were administered as intended. Effectiveness research, in contrast, evaluates the effectiveness of a treatment under conditions that more closely reflect the real world (Fritz & Cleland, 2003). Treatments evaluated in effectiveness research will often be compared to standard practice, and will be applied to more diverse populations than efficacy studies. However, because there is less

---

[3] Researchers sometimes refer to this issue as *transportability*.

stringent control on how the treatment is administered, effectiveness research makes sacrifices in terms of internal validity in exchange for greater generalizability (Fritz & Cleland, 2003). We will discuss efficacy and effectiveness research further in Chapter 15 when we discuss how to translate research findings into practice.

Experiments are usually conducted in areas where the phenomenon is fairly understood. For example, you need to know enough about a problem to develop a treatment that you believe will work. Other research designs such as qualitative research (see Chapter 6) are generally used when you begin exploration into a new area.

APPLICATION

Evaluating Internal Validity in Various Designs

When you are reading a research study, you should evaluate how strong the evidence is for internal validity. Confidence in internal validity will be highest for well-constructed experiments. However, a lot of psychotherapy research is nonexperimental (e.g., correlational data collected from a survey). Therefore, it is important researchers not overstate conclusions about cause and effect in nonexperimental research. Correlation does not mean causation due to the possibility of a spurious relationship. Even if a causal relationship exists, the direction of cause and effect may be unclear. A competent researcher will acknowledge these potential limits when discussing the results.

Evaluating the Quality of Experiments

There are a number of questions you can ask yourself when evaluating the quality of an experimental design (see also Appendix II). First, does the experiment include one or more comparison groups? Are the subjects randomly assigned to the groups? Both are necessary for an experiment to have strong internal validity. If the design is missing one of these ingredients, then the study may suffer from some of the threats to internal validity discussed in this chapter such as history, maturation, selection bias, or others. If the experiment was quasi-experimental and did not use randomization, the research should test to see if the groups are equivalent using pretest measures. Even if randomization was done, some studies may also measure the equivalence of groups on key measures, particularly if the number of subjects in the study was small.

Second, even if a randomized controlled study is used, are there other potential threats to internal validity? For example, is it possible the treatment improvement is due to a placebo effect? If alternative treatments are being compared, do differences in therapists across the groups pose a potential confounding factor? Likewise, is it possible that the threats listed in Table 3.1 have impacted the study? For example, does selective mortality create bias in favor or against the treatment? Many journals, especially those in the medical field, are requiring researchers to follow guidelines for reporting RCTs developed by the CONSORT Group (Moher et al. for the Consort Group, 2010; Schulz, Altman, & Moher for the CONSORT Group, 2010). These guidelines include providing a flowchart that documents the attrition of subjects throughout the phases of the study (recruitment, randomization, treatment, follow-up).

Third, were the treatments delivered as intended? For example, were the therapists properly trained in the approach? Often researchers will develop a manual for therapists to follow to ensure the treatment is delivered in a consistent manner. Stronger studies will also evaluate if therapists were faithful in adhering to the model.

Fourth, are there any concerns with how the effectiveness of the treatment was measured? Instruments used to measure outcomes should have good reliability and validity (see the previous chapter on measurement). Also, stronger studies often evaluate effectiveness using multiple outcome measures rather than rely on one indicator.

Fifth, what is the length of time over which the effectiveness was measured? Some studies measure the effectiveness only at the conclusion of treatment. Stronger studies will do a follow-up after a designated amount of time to see if the treatment gains are maintained over time. Superior studies will even do follow-ups of a year or more, although this tends to be the exception rather than the rule.

Sixth, are there factors that restrict the ability to generalize the findings of the experiment to the real world? This problem can arise if the research participants differ in an important way from those who will likely receive the treatment in the future. For example, excluding everyone who has suicidal ideation from a study intended to evaluate a treatment for depression limits the ability to generalize the findings. Problems can also arise if the treatment is delivered in a manner that is not likely to be feasible in the real world. Although the ability to generalize the findings is important, one must recognize that initial evaluations of a treatment will primarily focus on establishing efficacy or internal validity. Once the efficacy of a treatment has been established, then effectiveness studies can be designed to evaluate how successful the treatment is under more real-life conditions (see Chapter 15 for a more detailed discussion of efficacy and effectiveness research).

The Concept of Internal Validity in Therapy

Although clinicians seldom talk about internal validity, the concept is vitally important to psychotherapy. As therapists, we try to uncover the underlying causes (e.g., relationship patterns, psychopathology) to our clients' problems. This understanding is necessary to develop effective interventions. For example, rule-outs in psychopathology acknowledge that there may be more than one possible disorder to explain a client's symptoms, which parallels the concept of internal validity. Through further assessment, clinicians attempt to pinpoint an accurate diagnosis by eliminating other possibilities.

Like experiments, our interventions may help us confirm our hypotheses about the underlying problem. A child's positive response to a stimulant medication provides support that a child's behavioral issues are due to ADHD. However, like experiments, this only works if the therapist changes one thing at a time. If the therapist suggests more than one intervention at a time, the therapist will have a difficult time isolating what contributed to the change.

CHAPTER 4

External Validity and Sampling

Simone has been using emotionally focused therapy (EFT) with success with three recent couples. All three couples are heterosexual and have been married for more than 10 years. Simone is beginning to work with Taylor and Brent, a gay couple that have been together for 9 months. Conflict between the couple escalated after the couple began living together 3 months ago. Simone is wondering if EFT will be equally effective with this same-sex couple as with her heterosexual couples. She is also wondering if the length of the couple's relationship will impact its effectiveness. Although she may not think of it in these terms, Simone is asking questions about external validity.

External validity speaks to our ability to generalize findings from our research. In other words, can we confidently apply what we learned from our research to other people or settings? As this case example illustrates, external validity is highly dependent upon how the initial sample compares to the group in which we hope to generalize our findings. Therefore, external validity and sampling are intimately connected.

In this chapter, we will explore two general approaches to sampling called probability and nonprobability sampling. Although probability sampling methods offer better external validity, they can be difficult and expensive to do. In contrast, nonprobability sampling methods offer lower external validity but are usually easier and less costly to do. We will look more closely at the various ways of doing probability and nonprobability sampling and how they relate to external validity. In addition, we will examine how low response rates may negatively impact external validity if the individuals who choose to participate in a study are significantly different from those that do not.

THE BASICS OF EXTERNAL VALIDITY AND SAMPLING

External Validity

External validity refers to our ability to generalize our findings beyond our study. Our ability to generalize our findings is primarily determined by the sample of people we choose to study.[1] External validity will be strong if the sample of people we study is representative of the larger group of people to which we hope to generalize our findings.

Researchers use the term **population** to refer to the group (usually people) in which you would like to make your conclusions. Often this group is much larger than one can practically include in a research study (e.g., everyone voting in the next presidential election, all distressed couples, everyone who is depressed). Therefore, we usually study a subset of the general population called a **sample**. In some cases, it may be possible to study the entire population if it is small. It is feasible for a company with 100 employees to enroll everyone if it wants to evaluate worker satisfaction with the company's benefits.

Before talking further about sampling, it is important to note that external validity can be impacted by other factors than just who was studied. If the research context is significantly different from what would happen under normal circumstances, then this can impact external validity. For example, in the earlier chapter on experiments, we noted that pretesting could sensitize individuals to the treatment, thereby enhancing the treatment effect. Because individuals are rarely pretested outside of research, the magnitude of the treatment effect will not generalize to real-life conditions. In addition, if treatment conditions in a study are difficult to replicate in real life, then the treatment benefits may not extend beyond the research setting. Treatment studies where therapists are closely supervised and have small caseloads seldom mirror what clinicians typically experience in community agencies. If the effectiveness

---

[1] Because most studies focus on people, we will use this language. However, samples might be composed of things other than people, depending upon the nature of the study. An analysis of the family therapy literature, for example, might have a sample consisting of journal articles.

of the treatment is contingent on therapists having small case loads and strictly adhering to the treatment protocol, then the results may not generalize when put into practice in community agencies.

Sampling

The goal of sampling is to obtain a subset of the general population representative of the larger population in which we hope to generalize our findings. In order for a sample to be representative, individuals from the population should have an equal chance of being selected.[2]

Probability and nonprobability sampling are the two general approaches for creating a sample from the general population. **Probability sampling** has stronger external validity because everyone in the population has an equal chance or probability of being selected, resulting in a representative sample. In contrast, the likelihood or probability of individuals being selected from the general population is unknown when using **nonprobability sampling**. Because not everyone has an equal chance of being selected, people in the sample may not be representative of the population, resulting in lower external validity. However, nonprobability sampling is used in most studies, primarily because it can be considerably easier and less expensive to do. We will now examine the different ways to perform probability and nonprobability sampling.

Probability Sampling

In probability sampling, the sample is typically drawn from a list of the population called a **sampling frame**. Ideally, the sampling frame will include everyone in the population. Unfortunately, frequently it is difficult to get a list that perfectly aligns with the population (if one can even obtain a list at all). For example, a researcher studying the attitudes or practices of family therapists might use the membership list of the American Association for Marriage and Family Therapy (AAMFT) as the sampling frame. This list does not include all family therapists

---

[2]For the sake of simplicity, we have stated that everyone has an equal chance of being selected. Technically, it can also be an unequal chance provided the researcher knows what the probability is (e.g., there are twice as many males as there are females). It is essential that it be a known probability so that the researcher can weight each group accordingly to create a representative sample.

because some choose not to be members of AAMFT.[3] The researcher may be tempted to say the findings will generalize to all family therapists. However, we can only confidently generalize the results to members of AAMFT.

To ensure everyone has an equal chance of being included in the sample, researchers can use a variety of probability sampling methods to select individuals from the sampling frame. Using **simple random sampling**, all individuals are assigned a number, which are then randomly selected to create the sample. This approach is sometimes used when conducting telephone surveys. Computers can randomly generate phone numbers using a method called random digit dialing. These phone numbers are then used to determine who will be contacted for the telephone survey. Unlike using a phone directory, which does not contain unlisted numbers, random digit dialing ensures that every possible phone number has an equal chance of being selected.[4]

Systematic sampling creates a sample by starting at a random point in the list, and then choosing every nth person (e.g., every third person). For example, if you had a sampling frame of 1,000 individuals and you want a sample of 100 people, you would select every 10th person. Because systematic sampling typically delivers comparable results to simple random sampling and is often easier to do, it is more commonly used in practice.

In **stratified sampling**, the sampling frame or list is divided into strata or groups along important attributes (e.g., ethnicity/race, social class). Simple random sampling or systematic sampling is then used to fill each group or strata. Stratified sampling is used if the researcher wants greater assurance that the sample includes adequate representation of certain groups.

All three approaches require a sampling frame that contains a list of everyone in the population (or an approximation of it). However, a single list of the entire population does not always exist. In these situations, **multistage cluster sampling** may be the best alternative. Imagine you are interested in studying what percentage of undergraduate psychology students are interested in pursuing a graduate degree in family therapy. No list of the entire population of undergraduate psychology students

---

[3] Nearly half of family therapists live in California; many who do not belong to AAMFT.
[4] You may recognize that the sampling frame does not perfectly reflect the population because not everyone has a phone.

exists. However, it might be feasible to locate a list of all universities that offer undergraduate psychology degrees. From this list, you might select every fifth psychology program in the first stage of sampling. Next you would contact these programs to obtain a list of all their students. Every third student would then be randomly selected from each program's list to create our sample. Through this two-stage process, we will hopefully have created a representative sample of psychology students for our study.

Nonprobability Sampling

There are several types of nonprobability sampling, the most common being **convenience sampling**. This type of sampling is also referred to as *availability sampling, accidental sampling, haphazard sampling,* or *opportunity sampling.* In convenience sampling, the researcher uses a sample that is easily available.

Convenience sampling often has poor external validity for at least two reasons. First, individuals asked to participate in a study using this method are often not representative of the population. For example, a great deal of psychological research is conducted with undergraduate students because they are conveniently available to researchers in academic settings. However, undergraduate students are not representative of the general adult population in many ways, such as level of education, income, age, and marital status.

Second, researchers that seek volunteers through advertisements may introduce a bias in the sample through selection effects. A study that recruits engaged couples through newspaper announcements is probably more likely to attract highly motivated couples or couples experiencing distress.

One reason convenience sampling is so common is that it is cost effective. It can be difficult and expensive to obtain a sampling frame that is representative of a large population. Although concerns about external validity are high with convenience sampling, it is not always a fatal flaw. It may be acceptable to use convenience sampling if the researcher is doing exploratory work to determine if relationships exist between certain variables. Convenience sampling is often used in experimental studies where the primary focus is on internal validity rather than external validity. However, if the researcher is doing a survey to measure how prevalent certain attitudes or behaviors are, having a representative sample is critical to obtaining accurate results. Therefore, the type of sample that is required will depend upon the nature of the research questions.

Quota sampling attempts to improve on convenience sampling by making sure certain groups are adequately represented. For example, the researcher may specify that different racial or ethnic groups must represent a certain percentage of the sample. Quota sampling is similar to stratified sampling, except convenience sampling rather than probability sampling is used to fill each group. Therefore, the individuals may not be representative of that particular group when using quota sampling.

In **purposive sampling** (sometimes called **judgment sampling**), the selection of participants is guided by the researcher's judgment as to what type of cases will yield the best information to understand the phenomenon. The researcher may use selection criteria so that participants represent typical cases. For example, if Sofía is studying the impact of a family therapy training program on graduate students' well-being, she will attempt to find individuals representative of most students going through family therapy programs, who are typically young, single females. Or, the researcher may choose participants that are believed to cover the whole range of experiences. In this example, Sofía may want to select both male and female students, those that are single and married, or include individuals from different age groups. In some cases, the researcher may elect to find extreme cases or those that are atypical (sometimes called *deviant case sampling*) to better understand the phenomenon being studied. For example, Sofía may want to study students who dropped out of their training program to see what impact the program had on their well-being.

Purposive sampling is often used in qualitative research (see Chapter 6). In purposive sampling, external validity is established by comparing the study sample to the group in which you hope to apply the findings. If the new group is similar to the sample that was studied, then the results are likely to apply.

Sometimes researchers use a technique called **snowballing** to identify potential participants. Individuals who meet criteria for the study are asked to recommend others who may also fit the criteria. These individuals, in turn, may be able to identify others who fit the criteria, creating a snowballing effect. Snowballing may be used if individuals with a particular characteristic are difficult to locate or identify. For example, John and Montgomery (2012) used snowballing in a study that examined socialization goals of first-generation immigrant Indian families.

Response Rates

Researchers are seldom able to get everyone they select for their sample to participate in the study. They may not be able to contact some individuals, or others may be unwilling to participate. For example, if you select every fifth therapist from your local phone directory to study, it is unlikely you will be able to contact everyone because some may have recently retired, moved, or changed their number. Others may simply choose not to participate. The **response rate** is typically calculated by dividing the number of people who participated in the study by the number of people in the entire sample (which includes those that could not be reached or chose not to participate), and is often reported as a percentage.

Response rates can be important when evaluating studies such as surveys. Researchers who invest the money and effort to do probability sampling may end up with participants who are not representative if there is a low response rate. That is because individuals who chose to participate in a study may be very different from those who do not. For example, a clinic may send out a questionnaire to 1,000 clients served over the past 5 years to assess their satisfaction with therapy. If only 100 respond, then the response rate is 10%. It is possible that the 10% who responded are different from the 90% who did not. For example, it is conceivable that only those who were extremely satisfied or extremely dissatisfied were motivated enough to respond, leading to a sample that is not representative.

In some cases, researchers have preexisting information about everyone selected for the sample, which allows them to compare those who participated to those that did not. In the above example, the researcher could see if those who responded were different from those that did not on key variables such as type of therapy received (individual, couple, or family) or length of treatment. If those who responded are not significantly different from those that did not on key variables, then we have greater confidence the results will generalize to everyone.

In many cases, however, researchers do not have this information. Therefore, response rates are used to estimate this risk. It is assumed that the lower the response rate, the more likely it is that those who participated are different from those that did not.

What is an acceptable response rate? Babbie (2007) states that response rates above 50% are acceptable, above 60% are good, and those above 70% are very good. Some government agencies require that government funded surveys have a minimum response rate of 70% or above. However, a strong response rate does not guarantee that study participants are representative of the population. The 30–40% who chose not to respond may still be significantly different from those that did respond. However, a strong response rate usually means this is less likely to be the case.

Many studies have response rates well below 50% because researchers make only one appeal for individuals to complete a survey. To obtain good response rates, researchers typically have to send additional reminders or requests encouraging individuals to participate in the study. Offering incentives for participation can also improve the response rate. Stronger studies will put greater effort into increasing the response rate.

For nonprobability sampling methods, it is often not feasible to establish a response rate. Researchers sometimes advertise their studies through newspapers, the Internet, or word-of-mouth. In these cases, it is impossible to know how many people viewed the invitation to participate in the research, so one cannot calculate the percentage of those who responded. Again, confidence regarding external validity of studies conducted in this manner is typically low.

APPLICATION

Evaluating External Validity and Sampling in Research

Although evaluating external validity is most often associated with sampling issues, you should also evaluate the context in which the study results were obtained. Is the context different from what the normal context would be? If so, then this raises concerns regarding external validity.

Most concerns regarding external validity usually relate to sampling or who was studied. The fundamental question is whether the sample is representative of the population to which we hope to generalize the findings. To answer this question, you must first determine what is the population in which the researcher is hoping to generalize the findings. This is not always explicitly stated. Whether the sample is representative will depend upon how the population is defined. Some researchers may be tempted to overstate what can be generalized from their study, so pay careful attention to this issue.

There are several things to consider when evaluating the sampling procedures in a study. As a general rule, you can have greater confidence in a study that used probability sampling. However, you still need to evaluate if the sampling frame is representative of the population. As discussed, sampling frames are often not perfect matches with the population because a complete list of a population can be difficult to find or generate. Therefore, you must judge to what extent this creates a problem in terms of external validity.

In addition, you need to evaluate if a poor response rate has made the sample potentially unrepresentative. Ideally, the researcher will be able to analyze if responders are different from nonresponders to address this issue directly. Few studies, however, do this. Therefore, you must rely on the response rate to evaluate this risk. As stated earlier, 50% is generally acceptable, 60% is good, and 70% is very good. Although a strong response rate does not guarantee the sample is representative, it does significantly reduce the risk that nonresponders are different from responders.

If the researcher used nonprobability sampling, such as convenience or quota sampling, then there is a good chance the sample will not be representative of the population. That does not mean the results from the study cannot be of value, but one must be particularly cautious in generalizing the findings. The researcher should acknowledge this as a limitation of the study, and may even suggest ways in which the study participants could be different from those in the population. Be especially wary of researchers who do not address the limitations of using nonprobability sampling in their study.

For qualitative studies that use purposive sampling, evaluating external validity is different. Do you agree with the researcher's judgment regarding the criteria for selecting participants? For example, if the researcher attempted to find typical cases, do you think the criteria used achieved that result? Likewise, if the researcher was attempting to locate extreme or deviant cases, did the selection criteria fit this goal?

When attempting to apply findings from qualitative research to your own clinical work, you will need to compare the study sample with your clients. If there is a close match, then the findings are likely to generalize. If they do not match, then a good possibility exists that you will be unable to successfully apply them.

Building on this last point, you may have noticed that this is how you generalize the knowledge gained from your own clinical experience.[5]

---

[5]In Chapter 6, we will discover other ways in which the therapy process parallels doing qualitative research.

We often take what worked successfully with one client, and ask ourselves if those same ideas or interventions might work with another client with similar issues. The answer may depend upon how much the new client is like our earlier clients based upon a number of characteristics, such as gender, race/ethnicity, level of acculturation, religiosity or religious affiliation, sexual orientation, socioeconomic status, age, and others. If the new client is similar to the previous clients, then the ideas will likely generalize to the new case.

CHAPTER 5

Survey Research

Ashley meets Melissa and Donovan for their initial session. Melissa recently discovered that Donovan had an affair. Ashley asks Melissa, "How distressed have you been over the affair and have you seriously thought of divorce?" A researcher would have some concerns about Ashley's question. First, Ashley asked a closed-ended question that the client could simply answer by saying yes or no. It would be better to ask an open-ended question (particularly early in assessment) to encourage Melissa to describe her experience. Second, Ashley asked about two things in one question, which researchers call double-barreled. Melissa may have a difficult time answering the question if she wants to say yes to having experienced distress, but no to having had thoughts of divorce. Third, there is a risk that Ashley's question could be seen as suggesting that Melissa should be seriously considering divorce. As an alternative to the original question, Ashley might first ask Melissa, "How has the affair impacted you?" She might follow this up by asking, "How has the affair affected your feelings about the relationship?" If necessary, Ashley could ask more specific questions to clarify Melissa's answers.

In many ways, a clinical interview is similar to a survey that is orally administered. As a result, many of the considerations researchers use when designing survey questions are also applicable to our clinical work. Therefore, in addition to teaching you about surveys as a research methodology, we hope to strengthen your ability to ask good questions as a clinician.

Surveys are a powerful tool for collecting information. They allow us to access the private thoughts and feelings of individuals. In addition, surveys can help us learn about people's behaviors, particularly those that are done in private and difficult to observe. For survey information to be accurate, we rely on individuals to be honest, knowledgeable, and insightful, which are conditions that may not always be met. In addition, individuals must be cooperative in sharing their experiences. We will explore each of these considerations in more detail in this chapter.

Unlike other chapters, we will discuss more of the nuts and bolts of conducting survey research. That is because individuals who would never consider themselves researchers develop surveys all the time. For example, Lakeisha created a brief questionnaire so participants could evaluate the parenting workshop she had developed. The principles for conducting survey research can help us effectively collect information from individuals regarding their thoughts, feelings, preferences, opinions, or behaviors.

THE BASICS OF SURVEY RESEARCH

Advantages and Disadvantages of Survey Research

There are a number of advantages to **survey** research. First and foremost, surveys allow us access to the private thoughts, emotions, and behaviors of individuals that would be difficult or impossible to obtain otherwise. For example, we use surveys to measure people's perspectives or feelings on a wide variety of topics, ranging from politics to relationships. In addition, surveys allow us to ask about behaviors that would be hard to observe, such as sexual behavior.

Another advantage of surveys is that they can be used to predict the attitudes or behaviors of a large population based on a relatively small sample of people if appropriate sampling techniques are used (see Chapter 4). Samples in the low thousands, for example, have been able to reliably predict the outcome of general elections in the United States.

Surveys also offer information that is quantifiable. This makes the information easy to summarize. It also permits data to be analyzed using powerful statistical methods that can expand our understanding of the factors that relate to the phenomenon.

Surveys are also easily replicable. The same survey instrument can be administered at different points in time to see if behaviors or attitudes have changed. The same survey can also be given to different groups to allow comparisons to be made.

Surveys also have potential disadvantages. As stated above, a key strength of survey research is that it provides information on individuals' private thoughts, feelings, and behaviors. However, we rely on respondents to be honest, knowledgeable, insightful, and cooperative in sharing these things. Unfortunately, individuals may not always conform to these expectations. As discussed in Chapter 2, social desirability may lead individuals to be less than perfectly honest in their answers. They may overstate positive behaviors and underreport negative behaviors. If we ask individuals questions regarding topics in which they have little knowledge, then the information may be of questionable value. Some individuals may also lack insight, which may impair their ability to accurately identify what they are thinking or feeling. Finally, we rely on individuals to cooperate in participating in a study and answer our questions. However, this is not always the case because surveys often suffer from low response rates. Unfortunately, this creates problems in generalizing the findings if the individuals who respond to the survey are significantly different from those who do not.

Although the quantitative nature of surveys is an advantage in many regards, it may not offer the same richness of detail or insight that qualitative data can. Quantitative data based on closed-ended questions may tell you what attitudes individuals hold, but not necessarily why. Some researchers combine both closed-ended and open-ended questions, using qualitative methods to analyze the responses to open-ended questions. Therefore, surveys can be analyzed using both methods depending upon the nature of the questions.

Developing good surveys requires a basic knowledge of the topic. You need to know enough about an area to know what are good questions to ask. Therefore, surveys may not be the best approach for new areas of inquiry.

Another frequent limitation of surveys is that the data is frequently correlational in nature. As a result, there may be questions regarding cause and effect or internal validity (see Chapter 3). For example, because the variables on a survey are typically measured at the same time, the direction of cause and effect may be unclear if two variables are related.[1] In addition, there is the possibility that correlations are due to spurious relationships.

Although surveys can be used to accurately predict the attitudes or behaviors of a larger population based on a small sample, the accuracy of

---

[1] If surveys are administered to the same group of people over time, then it may be possible to determine cause and effect relationships since the temporal sequence may be known.

these results is highly dependent upon the sampling method used. Sometimes obtaining samples representative of the general population (see Chapter 4) can be costly or difficult to obtain. Often this type of research requires external funding to be feasible. Sometimes researchers can gain access to data sets other researchers or organizations have collected that are representative of the larger population. However, the analyses are limited to using the variables that the other researcher or organization collected, which may not be an ideal fit with what the researcher wants to study.

Types of Surveys

Surveys can take many forms. They can be orally administered by an interviewer either face-to-face or over the telephone. They can also take the form of written questionnaires that are completed on paper or electronically via the Internet. Each form offers advantages and disadvantages.

Face-to-face interviews typically have the highest response rate because the interviewer can establish rapport, and it is more interesting or engaging talking to someone than completing a questionnaire. Getting individuals to participate in telephone surveys is more challenging because individuals may question the legitimacy of the survey due to the pervasive presence of telemarketers.

Interviewers, whether face-to-face or through the telephone, can help respondents if they become confused or probe for further information when necessary. This makes them better suited for more complicated surveys. However, they are more expensive due to labor costs associated with using interviewers. This is particularly true for face-to-face interviews, which may include travel expenses for interviewers. Later we will also discuss how interviewers may introduce errors or a bias when collecting data if they are not properly trained.

Mail and Internet questionnaires typically cost less than face-to-face or telephone interviews. Questionnaires can also be completed anonymously, which may be critical for highly sensitive topics. However, questionnaires require that respondents be able to read. In recent years, questionnaires taken via the Internet are quickly replacing the traditional pencil and paper approach. Internet surveys are less expensive because they do not have printing or mailing costs. In addition, they can be done quickly because one does not have to wait for the questionnaires to be delivered or returned through the mail. However, Internet surveys require individuals to have access to computers and the Internet, as well as being comfortable using this technology.

Sampling issues may factor in what type of survey is used. Face-to-face interviews often mean collecting data locally. Logistically it is easier to do a national survey through telephone interviews, or using mail and Internet questionnaires. However, it may be difficult to obtain a list of mailing addresses or e-mails that is representative of the population one wishes to study. As described in Chapter 4, random digit dialing is a technique that some researchers use when conducting telephone surveys to create a probability sample of the general population. Random digit dialing circumvents the problem of using phone directories, which do not contain unlisted numbers.

The Basic Steps

Although there are some unique features between doing an interview and a questionnaire, the process of constructing an effective survey is the same in many regards. The first step is to define the **research questions,** which reflect the purpose of the study or what the researcher hopes to learn. Research questions are different from the questions asked in a survey because they are more global in nature (e.g., "Is there a relationship between marital satisfaction and level of differentiation?").

In the second step, the researcher decides what type of survey to use. This will be informed by a number of factors such as the purpose of the survey, the nature of the population being studied, and the resources available to the researcher. For example, a researcher interested in evaluating the extent to which community mental health services are used by the homeless living on the streets would require using face-to-face interviews because telephone interviews and mail/Internet questionnaires would not be feasible.

The next step is to write the actual survey questions. This step is critical because the quality of the questions determines the quality of the data. This process is so important that we will devote a separate section of this chapter to asking good questions.

When developing a survey, the researcher must consider how long it should be, which is based on a number of factors. Often the researcher is interested in collecting as much information as possible. However, the longer the survey, the less likely people will be to complete it. The topic of the survey is another determining factor. Individuals will invest more time completing a survey if the topic is both interesting and important to them. Finally, face-to-face interviews can also be longer because individuals enjoy the personal interaction of talking to an interviewer compared to the impersonal experience of completing a questionnaire.

Determining the order of survey questions is important. One reason is that the initial questions may influence whether the respondent completes the survey. Ideally the survey will begin with questions that are both interesting and easy to answer, which will engage the respondent. Questions that are difficult or threatening may discourage participation. For this reason, survey researchers typically avoid beginning surveys with demographic questions unless they are necessary to screen for eligibility. Demographic questions are not very interesting and are potentially threatening (e.g., asking about income or age).

The order of questions can also impact how they are answered because earlier questions provide a context for later questions. Survey questions often go from general to specific in a technique called **funneling**. Using this technique, you begin with more global questions, and then move to more specific questions. For example, when assessing marital happiness, you would first ask about overall satisfaction with the relationship before asking about specific areas, such as intimacy, sex, or communication. Asking about the specifics first may influence the global assessment of the relationship. If you first ask about certain areas where couples can experience conflict (e.g., sex, managing finances, division of household chores), then these answers may negatively color how the individual responds when asked about overall satisfaction.

In some cases, the order of the questions can be used to manipulate responses. A survey commissioned by the Public Broadcasting Service (PBS) began by asking about concerns relating to commercial broadcasting (Barnes, 1995), such as asking if the programming contained too much "violence and brutality." These questions preceded the critical question on whether federal funding should be increased for public broadcasting. Highlighting problems with commercial broadcasting first probably explains why respondents in the PBS survey were more supportive of using federal spending to subsidize public broadcasting than two other polls that looked at a similar question.

The order of questions also needs to make sense to the respondent so as to avoid confusion. When collecting historical information, it is best to ask questions in chronological order to avoid confusion. Questions should also be grouped by topic. Otherwise, skipping from topic to topic can confuse the respondent. Transitional statements are often used to mark a change from one topic to another.[2] For example, a survey might state, "That concludes the questions on your courtship. Now I am going to ask you some questions about your marriage."

Properly formatting the survey is an important task, particularly when designing questionnaires. A poorly formatted survey can lead to errors. For example, placing more than one question across a page may lead to the second question being overlooked (see Figure 5.1). Respondents (or interviewers) may also erroneously mark the wrong response box if they are placed horizontally rather than listed vertically (see Figure 5.1). Poorly formatted surveys can also discourage potential participants from completing a survey. A questionnaire with items crowded together and with small print may look intimidating, resulting in a lower response rate. Surveys that are professional in appearance will obtain a higher response rate than those that appear to be casually or carelessly designed.

Piloting (or pretesting) the survey is a critical but sometimes overlooked step. When piloting a survey, you ask individuals to complete the survey and give you feedback on what it was like to take it. It is best to pilot your survey with individuals who are similar to those who will be used in your study. Piloting can help you identify questions that are problematic or confusing so that they can be remedied before collecting data. Piloting can also help you determine how long it will take individuals to complete the survey.

Prior to beginning the study, telephone or face-to-face interviewers need to be trained to avoid introducing errors or biases when collecting the data. Interviewers learn how to properly record the data, and to ask questions in a uniform manner. If the interviewers must ask for additional information, they are instructed to do so in a manner that is neutral and does not lead the respondent (e.g., "Can you say more?"). Interviewers also must be careful not to subtly influence respondents, such as adding, "That is good," if they respond in a particular way.

1. What is your gender? Male ____ Female ____	2. What is your age? ____
3. Do you enjoy research? ____I love it ___ It is fun ___ It is OK ___ I dislike it ___ I hate it	

FIGURE 5.1. Examples of poorly formatted questionnaire items.

---

[2] A similar strategy is used when writing essays to transition between different ideas or paragraphs.

After collecting the data, the final steps are to analyze the data and report the findings. Descriptive statistics like means, frequency tables, or bar graphs can be powerful ways to summarize and communicate results (see Chapter 9). Inferential statistics using bivariate or multivariate statistics (Chapters 10 and 11) can be used to look for relationships between variables.

Asking Good Survey Questions

Questions can be either open-ended or closed-ended. **Open-ended questions** permit the respondent to answer in any way they like. An example of an open-ended question might be "What are your views on same-sex marriages?" This type of question is good for exploratory work because it allows the respondent to describe their experience in more detail and richness. However, the answers may be ambiguous, vague, or off-topic. Answers to open-ended questions can be difficult to analyze or summarize due to their narrative nature. Open-ended questions typically are better for interviews than questionnaires because people generally do not mind talking, but they often dislike writing.

Closed-ended questions offer the respondent choices from which to select. For example, when respondents are asked about their views of same-sex marriages, they might be offered the following choices: I approve of same-sex marriages, I disapprove of same-sex marriages, or I am undecided. The key advantage of closed-ended questions is that the answers are clear because they are preselected by the researcher. They are also easier to summarize and analyze. However, answers to closed-ended questions do not offer the same richness as open-ended questions, such as allowing respondents to state why they approve or disapprove of same-sex marriages.

The quality of data gained from closed-ended questions is only as good as the answer choices provided. Therefore, you need a sufficient knowledge of the topic to offer appropriate choices. Good survey questions must offer responses that are **exhaustive** by including all of the possible answers. One survey asked individuals to identify their race, but did not offer a choice for those who were biracial or multiracial. If the respondent is forced to choose only one answer, then the answers should be **mutually exclusive** so that only one answer applies. If you ask an individual to identify their marital status, the choices of single, married, and divorced are not mutually exclusive because a divorced individual is also single. Some would argue the question is also not exhaustive because it does not provide a category for cohabitating couples.

Researchers must also decide how many choices to provide respondents when using rating scales to measure intensity or degrees of an attribute (e.g., level of satisfaction, level of agreement or disagreement). Too many choices can overwhelm the respondent, particularly if the survey is being given orally. However, offering a small number of choices can reduce sensitivity, making it more difficult to distinguish differences between individuals. Another potential issue is whether or not to include a neutral category, like when asking individuals if they agree or disagree with a statement. Some advocate that most individuals are truly not neutral and should be forced to choose a position. Others believe a neutral category permits individuals without a strong preference to endorse an item that comes closest to their position. Some research suggests that the ratio of positive to negative is comparable regardless of whether or not a neutral category is offered (Bradburn, Sudman, & Wansink, 2004).

Asking clear questions requires paying attention to a number of factors. First, you may need to carefully operationalize or specify what you mean by certain words. If you ask about income, do you mean income before or after taxes? Do you mean the individual's income, or does it also include the total income for the household? Second, you must use words that are familiar and avoid using jargon. Some clients may not understand what you mean if you use clinical terms that are unfamiliar to people other than therapists. Your client may be perplexed, for example, if you ask her if she has an enmeshed relationship with her mother. Third, avoid double negatives. Potential confusion could arise if individuals are asked whether they agree or disagree with the following statement, "I am not in favor of mandatory premarital counseling for engaged couples." In this case, supporting mandatory counseling would require disagreeing with a negative statement. A more straightforward approach is to simply ask if the individual agrees or disagrees with the statement, "I am in favor of mandatory premarital counseling for engaged couples."

One must also avoid asking **double-barreled questions**, which inquire about more than one thing at a time. Asking if an individual favors mandatory premarital counseling and changing no-fault divorce laws to reduce divorce rates is an example of a double-barreled question. The individual may be confused on how to answer if they favor mandatory premarital counseling to reduce the divorce rate, but are not in favor of changing the divorce laws. This question should be split into two separate questions. The word *and* usually indicates a double-barreled question.

It is important to avoid **leading questions**, which encourage respondents to answer in a particular way, thereby biasing the results. Using emotionally charged words can create leading questions. The question "Do you favor eliminating discriminatory laws that prohibit same-sex marriages?" could be viewed as leading by using terms such as discriminatory or prohibit. In addition, questions can be leading based on the response choices that are provided. For example, a survey for evaluating therapy services is biased toward getting a satisfied response if the choices offered are *extremely satisfied, very satisfied, satisfied,* or *dissatisfied.*

The wording of questions can also influence how honest individuals will be, particularly because individuals normally want to appear socially desirable (see Chapter 2 on reactivity). Researchers can use a number of strategies to deal with social desirability. **Loading** questions can help reduce underreporting of negative behaviors (Bradburn et al., 2004). Loading prefaces the question with a statement that gives the respondent permission for engaging in a socially undesirable behavior. This may be done in a number of ways, such as acknowledging that everyone engages in the behavior: "Even the happiest couples sometimes argue. Did you and your partner argue at all last week?" Giving a reason for the undesirable behavior is another strategy used to load a question: "Many people find drinking alcohol helps them unwind. When is the last time you drank alcohol?" Loaded questions are different from leading questions in that they are used specifically to address underreporting of socially undesirable behaviors, whereas leading questions typically arise when assessing attitudes.

Another way to minimize underreporting of socially undesirable behavior is to presume the respondent engages in the behavior. Rather than first asking whether or not the individual drinks, you might ask, "How many drinks do you have each week?" When screening for HIV risk, one organization found that men were more likely to endorse having sexual activity with another man if they presumed the behavior ("What is the number of men with whom you have had sexual activity?"), rather than asking them first if they had ever been sexually active with another male.

Using the individual's language may also reduce social desirability (Bradburn et al., 2004). For example, when assessing for marijuana use, individuals might be asked what term they use for marijuana (e.g., weed), and then this term would be used in subsequent questions. Bradburn et al. (2004) also suggest that open-ended questions may reduce underreporting of socially undesirable behaviors. However, if you ask a closed-ended question it is important that you offer choices that are more extreme than the anticipated behavior. If you ask individuals how many beers they consume daily and your scale does not exceed five beers a day, then you will get an inaccurate picture if anyone drinks more than that. Individuals who drink five beers a day will also likely underreport the amount of drinking to avoid looking like they drink an extreme amount. However, if your scale goes up to 30 beers a day, then individuals may be more likely to acknowledge drinking five beers a day because it does not seem so unreasonable compared to drinking 20 or 30 beers a day.

Finally, **memory recall** is an important factor in asking questions. The time period over which the respondent is asked to recall things should match the importance of the event. You will be able to ask individuals to recall traumatic or important events (e.g., getting married, birth of child) that happened many years ago, but not what they had for dinner 1 week ago. Providing memory cues can enhance memory recall. For example, if you asked therapists which social networking sites they belong to, you might get a more complete list by including possible examples (e.g., Facebook, LinkedIn, Twitter). Having individuals keep records or diaries can also aid in recall, particularly for daily events.

APPLICATION

Evaluating Survey Research

To properly evaluate survey research, you will ideally be able to inspect the actual survey. Unfortunately, researchers seldom include the survey in a journal article. If you do have access to the survey, then you will want to inspect the questions to make sure they are properly written. For example, you will want to make sure the questions are not confusing, double-barreled, or leading in some manner. You will also want to evaluate the response categories to ensure they are mutually exclusive (if applicable), exhaustive, and provide sufficient sensitivity based on the number of choices. It is also helpful to examine the order of the questions and their formatting (for questionnaires) because they can influence how respondents answer the questions.

If you do not have access to the actual survey, you must rely on other indicators that the researcher is competent, such as how other methodological issues are addressed (e.g., sampling, statistical analysis, appropriate conclusions drawn regarding internal and external validity). Some surveys include previously developed scales as part of the survey instrument, which may provide greater confidence in the survey. However, there should be evidence for the reliability and validity of these scales as discussed in Chapter 2. You can also have greater confidence if the researcher states the survey was piloted or interviewers were trained (if applicable). Unfortunately, this is often not made explicit.

The issues we discussed in the previous chapter on external validity and sampling are particularly salient for survey research. It is important to evaluate if the sample is representative of the population. For example, what type of sampling method was used (probability, nonprobability), and how does this impact your confidence in the external validity of the findings? You should also remember a low response rate could impact how representative a sample is. Therefore, it is important to consider what kind of response rate was achieved, or if the researcher compared respondents to nonrespondents to determine if they were significantly different in some way. If there are concerns about external validity, the researcher should comment on this in the discussion.

Due to the correlational nature of most survey research, it is difficult to determine cause and effect. It may be difficult to know either the direction of causality, or if a spurious relationship exists. Therefore, you need to evaluate if the researcher is sensitive to potential issues regarding internal validity.

Developing Surveys

There may be situations where you will want to develop your own survey. For example, a survey could be developed to assess client satisfaction with your services. Or, you might develop an intake form for your clients to complete prior to starting therapy. Using the tools and principles we described in this chapter will permit you to construct an effective survey instrument.

Asking Questions

Guidelines for developing effective survey questions (e.g., avoid jargon, avoid double-barreled questions) can easily be applied to asking effective clinical questions. Like researchers, we must confront the issue of social desirability as clinicians. How we ask questions (e.g., loading the question, presuming the behavior, the choices for answers we offer) can impact how honest our clients will be. Offering confidentiality also encourages greater honesty. Therefore, many of the tools that survey researchers use are also at our disposal as clinicians.

CHAPTER 6

Qualitative Research

The two designs we have discussed so far (experimental research and survey research) are quantitative methodologies because they use numbers to understand a phenomenon. In contrast, qualitative studies use words to understand a phenomenon. Therefore, qualitative research is a good approach to use when trying to understand how individuals experience things (e.g., family life, therapy), particularly if one wants to know the meaning they attribute to these experiences. Qualitative research is also good when exploring a new area of investigation because description is often the first step toward understanding a phenomenon.

Qualitative research can take many different forms, which we will discuss in this chapter. In the family therapy field, qualitative research frequently involves conducting interviews with individuals or with focus groups. These interviews are typically transcribed and analyzed to uncover patterns, themes, or new insights.

Although differences exist between the various approaches to doing qualitative research, they also share much in common. Therefore, we will be able to describe key considerations for conducting and evaluating qualitative research that can be applied across a diverse range of approaches. We will conclude the chapter by looking at the strong parallels between how qualitative research and therapy are conducted.

THE BASICS OF QUALITATIVE RESEARCH

What Is Qualitative Research?

Qualitative research refers to a variety of designs that can be used to study a phenomenon. Qualitative approaches share some commonalities that distinguish them from **quantitative research**. First, qualitative research relies on description or words to understand a phenomenon. In contrast, quantitative research collects or transforms data into numerical form, which permits analysis using statistical techniques.

Qualitative research is frequently used to generate new insights or hypotheses. This distinguishes it from quantitative research, which is often used to test preexisting hypotheses. Thus, qualitative research is often seen as exploratory rather than confirmatory in nature. This is consistent with the descriptive nature of qualitative research because the first step in understanding a phenomenon is often to describe it.

Qualitative research is **inductive** in nature, going from specific to general. Qualitative research derives generalities in the form of patterns, themes, or theoretical models from data. For example, a researcher might interview family therapists in training programs to explore what factors impact emotional well-being. The researcher goes in with no preconceived hypotheses. However, through carefully analyzing the statements (data) made by the therapists, the researcher begins to uncover patterns or themes that are consistent across the different interviews. As a result, a new understanding of factors that can impact the emotional well-being of therapists in training programs has emerged.

In contrast to qualitative research, quantitative research frequently follows a **deductive** process, going from general to specific.[1] The researcher takes a theory (general) and derives or deduces specific hypotheses from it. Studies are then designed to generate data to test these hypotheses. For example, the researcher who studied factors that predict emotional well-being among therapists in training programs may follow up the qualitative study with a quantitative one. In this study, she may have specific hypotheses that she is trying to confirm, such as emotional well-being is positively related to self-care. To test this hypothesis, she will give therapists instruments that measure their emotional well-being and frequency of self-care activities. If the scores strongly correlate with one another, then she has confirmed her hypothesis.

---

[1]Categorizing all quantitative research as purely deductive is an oversimplification because quantitative research can be used both for confirmatory or exploratory purposes.

Finally, qualitative researchers tend to see reality as more subjective than objective. Qualitative researchers typically believe that what we see and believe is shaped by our social context. Thus, qualitative researchers are often interested in the meaning that individuals ascribe to what is happening in their lives. In this regard, qualitative research is consistent with a narrative approach to therapy.

There are a number of ways to do qualitative research. One of the most common ways in which qualitative research is done in the family therapy field is through **in-depth interviews**. Participants are asked to share their experience regarding a particular topic, such as infertility, parenting children with special needs, affairs, or even clients' experiences of therapy. Research of this nature can be an example of a type of research called **phenomenology**.[2] Phenomenological research seeks to understand how individuals make meaning out of their personal experiences (Dahl & Boss, 2005). For example, Hall and Sandberg (2012) used a phenomenological methodology to study African Americans who overcame barriers to participate in family therapy. Through this exploratory study, participants identified a number of barriers they faced (e.g., stigma attached to therapy, affordability), as well as some of the factors that helped them overcome the barriers.

In-depth interviews may vary in terms of how structured they are. In structured interviews, everyone is asked all of the same open-ended questions. At the opposite end of the continuum, the interview may be quite unstructured and conversational in nature, with the participant having a lot of discretion over the direction of the conversation. Often semi-structured interviews are used, which falls between the two extremes. Using a semi-structured approach, the interviewer is expected to cover certain topics, but attempts to make the interview as conversational as possible within this structure. The interviews are typically recorded, transcribed, and then analyzed to describe or generate new insights about the phenomenon.

Another common way in which qualitative research is conducted is through the use of **focus groups**, which gathers individuals together to discuss a particular topic (Piercy & Hertlein, 2005). In a study conducted by the first author, students and supervisors were brought together in focus groups to explore experiences with self-disclosure on the part of supervisors (Williams & Dombeck, 1999). An advantage of focus groups

---

[2] Although phenomenological research relies heavily on personal interviews, it may also include other forms of data collection (e.g., personal observation, studying artifacts).

is that comments from group members may stimulate additional thoughts for others, thereby leading to a richer discussion. However, a potential disadvantage is that individuals may be hesitant to offer perspectives that are different from the majority. Like in-depth interviews, focus groups are typically recorded, transcribed, and the content analyzed using qualitative methods described later in the chapter.

A number of other qualitative methods exist, although they are less frequently used in family therapy research. **Ethnography**, which grew out of the field of sociology and anthropology, is the study of cultures or social groups. The ethnographer becomes immersed in the culture or setting being studied. Insights about the social group are obtained through observation, interviews, or analyzing documents and other cultural artifacts (e.g., newspapers, letters). Ethnographers take extensive notes based on their observations, which become part of the data that is analyzed. Tubbs and Burton (2005) describe an ethnography that was done to better understand parenting practices in low-income, urban families. Semi-structured interviews were conducted with mothers within these families. Researchers also observed the families by accompanying the mother and her children when they would visit the doctor, welfare office, or other places.

In an **autoethnography**, the focus is on the researcher's personal experiences, with the goal of providing a reflexive account of the researcher's life and how it relates to his or her culture. One example was a study by six family therapists who used an autoethnography approach to describe their experiences working in a child welfare program designed for family reunification (Jager et al., 2009). The therapists shared lessons they learned, such as the need to advocate for disempowered families, the importance of cultural competence, and increasing effectiveness through collaboration between therapists, social services, and the courts.

Dialogue between individuals can also be analyzed using a qualitative approach called **conversation analysis** (Gale, 1996). The conversation or dialogue between individuals is recorded and analyzed to gain insight into the dynamics of the relationship, such as between a therapist and client. In one study, Sutherland and Strong (2011) used conversation analysis to examine how Karl Tomm, a noted family therapist, attempted to create collaboration with a couple in a therapy session. For example, one way that Karl Tomm tried to establish collaboration was to downgrade his expert status, such as offering his insights tentatively, or using language that suggested his comments were observations rather than objective truths. This, in turn, invited the clients to provide feedback on his comments, which the authors labeled reciprocal editing.

Qualitative methods can also be used to study recorded communication, such as publications within a field. For example, Bischoff, Springer, Felix, and Hollist (2011) did a qualitative analysis of 15 published case studies to identify the key themes that characterized medical family therapy. One of the key themes was recognizing the importance of attending to a client's experience of disease from a biological, psychological, social, and spiritual perspective. In the next chapter, we will discuss how a content analysis of recorded communication can also be done using quantitative methods.

Strengths and Limitations of Qualitative Research

Some researchers have debated the relative merits of qualitative and quantitative research in an evidence-based approach. Our view is that both qualitative and quantitative designs have merit, and one must match the methodology to the type of research questions being asked. We will discuss this issue further in Chapter 12 when we describe our approach to evidence-based practice.

Qualitative research has several strengths, which makes it ideal for certain purposes. Since the first step to understanding a new phenomenon is often to describe it, qualitative research's emphasis on description is a good fit when exploring a new area. In addition, one may not necessarily know in advance what is important to study when investigating a phenomenon for which little is known. Qualitative research gives the researcher the flexibility to change the focus of inquiry based on what insights begin to emerge.

Qualitative research is also suited to exploring the meaning that people ascribe to experiences in their lives. Qualitative research typically seeks to understand experiences from the participant's perspective (sometimes referred to as the insider's perspective) rather than testing the researcher's hypotheses or framework (the outsider's perspective). The use of words rather than numbers can make it easier to capture the nuances that are necessary to fully understand the meaning of individuals' experiences.

Qualitative research can also provide a more holistic picture of a phenomenon, which allows one to consider multiple factors simultaneously. Thus, some believe qualitative research is a better fit with a systems orientation and is ideal for studying complex processes such as therapy or family processes.

However, the holistic approach to qualitative research presents some challenges when addressing questions around cause and effect. With so many variables operating simultaneously, it is hard to establish internal validity. Unlike experiments, qualitative research lacks the necessary control of variables that allows us to determine with certainty cause-and-effect relationships.

Qualitative research can also present challenges when generalizing findings to a larger population. Qualitative studies can help the researcher identify important attitudes, experiences, or behaviors that may be found within a population. However, due to small samples and nonprobability sampling, qualitative research cannot tell us the percentage of individuals within the general population who think, feel, or behave in that manner. Survey research using probability sampling is best suited for answering these questions.

Qualitative and quantitative methods can complement each other. Qualitative research may be used initially to explore a new area, with subsequent studies incorporating quantitative designs. For example, the Center for Marriage and Family initially studied couples with different religious backgrounds using qualitative research because little was known about these couples other than their increased risk for marital distress. Focus groups and in-depth interviews helped the research team learn more about the rewards and challenges interchurch couples faced (Williams & Lawler, 2000). These insights helped the team develop a survey instrument that was administered using a national, probability sample (Center for Marriage and Family, 1999).

Some studies simultaneously collect quantitative and qualitative data because they offer different types of information. A study that use a combination of quantitative and qualitative approaches is sometimes called **mixed methods research**. For example, a survey may contain both closed-ended and open-ended questions. The closed-ended questions provide numerical findings (means, percentages, etc.) that can quantify certain aspects of the phenomenon. However, open-ended questions can add qualitative data that can fill in our understanding of what the numbers mean, such as why respondents endorsed particular attitudes or behaviors.

Key Considerations in Doing Qualitative Research

There are several important features when it comes to designing and conducting qualitative research. These features can be applicable to a variety of qualitative designs.

Define the Purpose of the Study

The first step is for the researcher to define the purpose of the study. The researcher will need to decide if a qualitative approach is the best design based on the purpose of the study. In the supervisor self-disclosure study mentioned earlier (Williams & Dombeck, 1999), the exploratory nature of a qualitative design was deemed appropriate because there was no existing literature on the topic.

Develop Guiding Research Questions

After defining the purpose, it is important to develop guiding research questions, which provide direction to the researcher on where to explore. In the supervisor self-disclosure study (Williams & Dombeck, 1999), the primary guiding research questions were:

1. "What are the potential benefits to supervisors using self-disclosure?"
2. "What are the potential risks to supervisors using self-disclosure?"
3. "What are possible guidelines supervisors can use for the appropriate use of self-disclosure?"

Guiding research questions can change or evolve as the researcher learns more about the phenomenon through collecting and analyzing data.

Define the Participants and the Setting

The researcher must also define who will be studied. Like quantitative research, this decision will be informed by the purpose and guiding research questions. In the supervisor self-disclosure study, the decision was made to interview both supervisors and student trainees because it was thought that they might have different perspectives. As we described in Chapter 4, qualitative studies typically rely on purposive or judgment sampling. The researcher selects individuals that will offer the best insight into the phenomenon. In some cases, this may mean selecting people who are typical. It may also include trying to find a range of experiences, or perhaps even searching for individuals who are exceptions or extreme examples.

External validity in qualitative research is established by comparing the study sample to another group to which you hope to generalize the findings. If they are similar, then the findings will most likely generalize.

Therefore, qualitative researchers should carefully describe the sample they used so the reader can determine how similar or different the sample is to the group in which he or she wants to apply the findings.

Ethnographers also need to define what setting they used to observe and study groups. Where the research is conducted may have implications for who and what is observed. For example, a researcher's observations about the homeless may be different if individuals who live on the streets are studied rather than those who live in transitional housing.

Define the Researcher's Perspective

Qualitative researchers believe that who the researcher is may influence how the data is analyzed and interpreted. Therefore, qualitative researchers will describe their background and theoretical perspective so the reader can appreciate how this might inform data collection and analysis. Researchers will obviously want to state what formal theory they are using because it will influence their perspective. For example, a researcher with training in cognitive-behavioral therapy will more likely focus on the thought processes when studying couple dynamics, whereas a researcher with an emotionally focused background will more likely be attuned to the couple's emotional experiences. Our personal beliefs, values, and experiences can also influence our perspective. Therefore, qualitative researchers will ideally describe their background (e.g., training, gender, race/ethnicity) so the reader can determine if it may have created a particular lens from which the researcher viewed the data.[3] For example, it would be important to know if the researcher was male or female in a study that examined gender issues in therapy because gender socialization could potentially influence the researcher's perspective.

Define the Researcher's Role

The researcher must also define what role or relationship they will have with the research participants. This is particularly important in ethnographic research. Ethnographers must decide if they will be a participant or simply an observer. Being a participant may allow researchers to gain special insights because they are sharing similar experiences with the people they are studying.[4] Being a participant may also help build rela-

---

[3] In Chapter 8 we will discuss further the role of values in research.

[4] This is why many therapists believe that having been in therapy themselves is helpful because it can give them better insight into what it is like to be a client.

tionships with the people you are studying, which in turn may allow you to obtain privileged information that would have been difficult to obtain otherwise. For example, Babbie (1992, pp. 303–304) describes how a graduate student named Randy Alfred set out to study the Church of Satan. Through his feigned conversion, Alfred eventually became appointed to the ruling body of the Church of Satan as its official historian. Thus, Alfred was able to gain privileged access to important documents and top members of the Church, including its leader Anton LaVey. As a result, Alfred was able to gain important information and insights he might not otherwise have been able to obtain if he were simply an outside observer.

However, there are potential risks to being a participant. The researcher's participation may change the group or process that is being studied. In addition, the risk of losing objectivity becomes greater as the researcher becomes more involved. Some anthropologists, for example, have become so enamored with the cultures they were studying that they became part of the culture, referred to as "going native."

Researchers must also consider the extent to which they will be concealed or nonconcealed observers. If you are a concealed observer, then you are less likely to influence or alter the behavior of the people you are studying. However, being a concealed observer may present some ethical issues because individuals are unable to give voluntary and informed consent to being in the study (see Chapter 8 for a discussion of ethical issues in research). Unless you are observing people in public, issues of privacy may also arise.

Regardless of the type of qualitative research, preexisting relationships between the researcher and participants could influence the study. In the supervisor self-disclosure study, the primary researcher was careful not to interview students he was supervising at the time. Otherwise, the supervisor–trainee relationship could have impacted how honest the trainees would have been in discussing their experiences.

Define the Types of Data That Will Be Collected

Interviews are an important part of most qualitative studies, particularly within family therapy. Some qualitative studies rely exclusively on interviews. Sometimes researchers interview informants, who are individuals that may be able to offer additional insights about the group being studied. In therapy, parents and teachers can be informants used to better understand children. Typically, interviews are recorded so that they can be transcribed and then analyzed.

Qualitative researchers, particularly ethnographers, may collect other forms of data in addition to interviews. Ethnographers often observe people or events, and then write detailed notes describing what they observed. These notes then become part of the data. They may also collect artifacts such as letters, photos, memos, newspapers, videos, or other materials that may give insight into the culture or phenomenon being studied.

Define How the Data Will Be Analyzed

In contrast to quantitative research, qualitative researchers do not wait until all the data is collected to begin analysis. Qualitative researchers collect and analyze data concurrently because they may not know what the most important thing to study is when exploring a new area. Therefore, qualitative researchers need the freedom to go where the data takes them.

As stated earlier, analysis of qualitative data is an inductive process. The **constant comparative method** is frequently used in analyzing qualitative data. Using this approach, the researcher continually sorts and categorizes new observations, which over time results in an emerging framework for understanding the phenomenon (Echevarria-Doan & Tubbs, 2005).

Using the constant comparative method, the researcher begins by coding the data, which requires going through a transcript line by line and identifying the key concepts or ideas. Figure 6.1 shows a section of transcript from the supervisor self-disclosure study that was coded. You will notice that only one key idea may be expressed in a long passage, whereas in other cases, an idea may be expressed in a single sentence.

During the analysis, similar ideas are grouped together into categories. As the researcher goes through the transcript, he or she determines if the idea belongs in an existing category, or if it requires a new category. In addition to adding new categories, existing categories may be changed or refined as new insights emerge from the analysis. The researcher may also create broader, more abstract categories that contain specific subcategories. For example, in the supervisor self-disclosure study, categories were created for each of the ways in which supervisor self-disclosure could impact trainees. These categories were eventually put into two broader categories that reflected the potential benefits and risks of supervisor self-disclosure.

In some cases, the researcher may seek out new cases to provide

Transcript

Interviewer: Are there other reasons for or against self-disclosure?

Male supervisor A: I think someone mentioned this before, but I think it has the potential of normalizing things. I think that I have used it for a normalizing function—say "I've experienced it too." Or to demonstrate frustrations with clinical work, how I've succeeded with clinical work. I think all of those things can have a normalizing function, and I think that is an upside to self-disclosure. **[1]** I think that it can also be modeling on how to self-disclose—that you could be a positive answer. **[2]**

Male supervisor B: I think the downside is you get a merging in the relationship that is not appropriate to a professional relationship, and it either becomes too friendly or too sexual. **[3]** There isn't the ability for the supervisee to respond to an authority figure. **[4]**

Female supervisor: The only other thing that I could think of is that sometimes I think that if I went too far in self-disclosure, I would really be wasting my supervisee's time because they may not want to hear it. **[5]** The supervision is for them, and they may not want to hear all my personal stories. **[6]**

Coding of Transcript

[1]—This passage was placed in the category "Self-disclosure can normalize a trainee's experience."

[2]—This sentence was placed in the category "Self-disclosure can model how to appropriately self-disclose."

[3]—This sentence was placed in the category "Self-disclosure can create a relationship that is professionally inappropriate."

[4]—This sentence was placed in the category "Self-disclosure can result in loss of authority for the supervisor."

[5]—This sentence was placed in the category "Self-disclosure can take time away from other supervision priorities."

[6]—This sentence was placed in the category "Self-disclosure should be done with the trainee's needs in mind."

FIGURE 6.1. Sample coding of transcript excerpt.

additional insight into the phenomenon. If the researcher chooses cases to help in developing an emerging theory, then this is often referred to as **theoretical sampling**.

Ideally, qualitative researchers will continue to collect and analyze data until they reach a condition called **saturation**. Saturation occurs when analysis of new cases does not yield any new insights. Analysis of additional cases simply repeats themes or insights found in earlier cases.

During data analysis, patterns or themes begin to emerge. Qualitative researchers will often write memos[5] to themselves to articulate these patterns or themes as they discover them. Eventually these patterns or themes can be formulated into an **analytical framework** for describing or understanding a phenomenon. In our example (Williams & Dombeck, 1999), analyses of focus group data led to the discovery of several potential benefits to supervisor self-disclosure (e.g., normalizing a therapist's struggles, modeling of appropriate self-disclosure), as well as potential risks (e.g., take time away from supervision, putting focus on supervisor's needs). Guidelines that supervisors could follow to minimize the potential risks of using self-disclosure also emerged from the study. For example, there should be a clear clinical purpose behind a supervisor's self-disclosure, and the supervisor should only disclose material they have properly worked through.

An analytical framework can take many forms. For example, it may be a set of new hypotheses about the phenomenon. Or, it might be a taxonomy or classification system for describing the phenomenon, such as classifying parenting styles as either authoritarian, authoritative, or laissez-faire. At higher levels of abstraction, the relationship between concepts may be formulated into a theory. This process of building a theory inductively from qualitative data is called developing a **grounded theory** (see Echevarria-Doan & Tubbs, 2005; Strauss & Corbin, 1998).

Develop Trustworthiness

Qualitative researchers have developed a number of different techniques to ensure the accuracy or trustworthiness of their findings. One common approach is to use **triangulation,** which requires the researcher to collect information from multiple sources to crosscheck the findings. Greater confidence can be placed in the validity of the findings if they are consistent across different sources.[6] Getting the perspective of both trainees and supervisors was one way in which the data was triangulated in the supervisor self-disclosure study.

Prolonged engagement is another way to ensure trustworthiness of the findings, which requires the researcher spend sufficient time within

---

[5] These memos are sometimes referred to as *theoretical memos*, particularly if the researcher is attempting to build a theory from the analysis.

[6] Journalists often seek a second or third source to confirm a fact or story, which is a form of triangulation.

a culture or social setting to fully understand it. This is especially important in ethnographic research, and helps ensure that key aspects of the phenomenon have not been missed or overlooked.

Member checking is another approach that can be used. The researcher's findings are shared with the research participants prior to publication to confirm they accurately reflected their experiences. Finally, **peer debriefing** can be used to confirm the findings. A professional colleague independently reviews the data and coding to determine if he or she would reach a similar conclusion.

Write Up the Results

Qualitative results are presented in a manner different from quantitative research. Rather than presenting tables of numbers or statistical results, a qualitative researcher describes the analytical framework that emerged from the data. The qualitative researcher includes quotes or narrative descriptions that illustrate and provide support for the conclusions. For example, the following quote was used in the supervisor self-disclosure study to show how supervisors can help normalize the struggles of being a beginning therapist through their own self-disclosure (Williams & Dombeck, 1999, p. 24). One student stated, "When the supervisors talk about similar experiences with clients, and you hear their mess-ups, it gives you an idea that—'OK, this is part of the growth process and I'll get over this hump.'" These narratives are sometimes called **rich–thick descriptions** because they may provide a detailed description of the phenomenon.

APPLICATION

Evaluating Qualitative Research

The above steps suggest questions you can ask yourself when evaluating a qualitative study (see also Appendix II). First, was the purpose of the study clearly defined? Does it seem to be a good fit with a qualitative methodology? Ideally, the researcher will also articulate the guiding research questions that provided additional focus for the inquiry.

Second, were the participants in the study clearly described? This will be important for evaluating if the findings will generalize to another group. The researcher should also clearly describe the setting in which an ethnography was done.

Third, was the researcher's background and frame of reference clearly described? This should include any theoretical perspective that informed the researcher's work. In addition, a good qualitative researcher will describe other experiences or attributes that could potentially influence interpretation of the data. This will help you evaluate if the researcher's background may have introduced a bias.

Fourth, did the researcher clearly define the role he or she had in the study? For qualitative studies that included observation, it will be important for the researcher to describe the extent to which he or she was a concealed observer. If the researcher was not concealed, did individuals behave differently knowing they were being observed? Was the researcher strictly an observer, or did he or she interact with the participants in some manner? If the researcher was a participant, what are the potential benefits and risks to the study? What type of relationship, if any, did the researcher have with the participants prior to or during the study, and how might this impact the study?

Fifth, did the study clearly describe what type of data was collected and how it was obtained? For most studies within family therapy, interviews will be the primary method of data collection, which are typically transcribed for data analysis.

Sixth, did the research clearly specify how the data were analyzed? Did they use an established method (e.g., constant comparative method) to analyze the data? Ideally, the study will provide a clear description of how the data were analyzed. Did the researcher state if saturation was reached? If not, it is possible new findings would have emerged if additional cases were analyzed.

Seventh, did the research describe the methods used to improve the trustworthiness of the data (e.g., triangulation, member checking)? The more methods employed, the greater confidence one can have in the findings.

Finally, did the study include quotes or narratives (e.g., rich–thick descriptions) to support the analytical framework? Do the quotes or descriptions support the researcher's conclusions?

Qualitative studies of high quality should address all of these issues. Any study that does not address one or more of these issues or does so in a cursory manner should be viewed in a more cautious manner.

How Qualitative Research Parallels Clinical Work

One could easily argue that a clinician operates like a qualitative researcher with each case, particularly in the early assessment phase of therapy. In the beginning, both the researcher and the clinician must define the purpose of their work. For the clinician, this means defining the goals for therapy.

Once goals are established, the clinician attempts to learn as much as possible about the clients' experience of the problem and why it exists. "Guiding research questions" can help guide this exploration, which might include:

"What is the nature of the problem?"
"What solutions have been attempted?"
"What strengths or resources do the clients possess?"
"Are there mental health disorders that must be ruled out?"
"How do family members interact around the problem?"

Defining who will be in therapy parallels the researcher's need to define who will be studied. If a parent brings in a child as the identified patient, will the therapist only work with the child? Or, will the therapist decide the whole family needs to be included to properly understand the child's behavior? The therapist must also define in what settings the clients will be assessed. Is it sufficient to simply observe the child in the therapy office, or will it be helpful to observe the child in other settings such as the classroom?

Like qualitative researchers, therapists need to be aware of how their background or perspectives can influence what information is collected and how it is interpreted. The theoretical orientation of a therapist will obviously impact what they look for during assessment. A structural family therapist may look for different things than a therapist working from a narrative or Bowen perspective. Other factors, such as personality, values, life experiences, gender, or cultural background (to name a few), may also come into play. Being aware of how these factors influence one's therapy may reduce the likelihood of having blind spots or biases.

In qualitative research, the researcher's role can influence the process (e.g., observer vs. participant, concealed or nonconcealed). This is also true for therapists. Our clients may try to be on their best behavior in the beginning of therapy, knowing they are being observed. As therapists, we are both a participant and an observer of the process. Through our questions, we may be changing the very process we are attempting to assess (e.g., through reactivity). Fortunately, our questions may change the interactions in positive ways by introducing new perspectives. As therapists, we also risk being inducted into the family dynamics through a parallel or isomorphic process, a form of "going native."

Similarities also exist between the qualitative researcher and the therapist because both collect and analyze data simultaneously, going where the data takes them. The goal in qualitative research and therapy is to develop an analytical framework that is inductively derived from the data. In a family therapy context, the therapist listens to the clients' stories and observes their behavior. On the basis of this content (data), the therapist attempts to identify the client's process (analytical framework). For example, a therapist working with a couple may identify a cycle or pattern with which the couple struggles.

Improving the trustworthiness of the findings is also important to therapists. Anyone who has worked with couples knows the importance of getting each partner's perspective to get an accurate picture of the relationship, which can be viewed as a form of triangulation. One of the benefits of working with families or couples is that triangulation is naturally built into the process. However, we can employ other methods to strengthen trustworthiness. When we share our conceptualization with the clients to see if they are in agreement with our formulations, we are using something similar to member checking. We can also use peer consultation and supervision as a form of peer debriefing.

Finally, as we discussed in Chapter 4 on external validity, therapists generalize the findings from one case to another much in the same way that qualitative researchers decide if the findings will apply to another sample. Many therapists believe that conducting research is very different from doing clinical work. However, the many similarities between clinical work and qualitative research challenge this view.

CHAPTER 7

Miscellaneous Research Designs

The designs we have studied so far are some of the most frequently used in family therapy research. In terms of the toolbox of research designs, these would be equivalent to the hammer, screwdriver, and wrench. However, depending upon the nature of the job or research question, sometimes other tools or designs are necessary. Therefore, before we transition to talking about ethics and statistics in research, we will explore a diverse range of research designs you are likely to encounter at some point.

We will begin by describing meta-analysis, a design that can be used in place of a literature review to summarize results from multiple studies (most often experiments). We will also look at reversal (ABA, ABAB) and multiple-baseline designs. These designs can be used instead of experiments to test the effectiveness of a treatment using very small samples. Next we will discuss two different designs that use coding systems as part of their design—content analysis and observational research. Content analysis focuses on coding recorded media (e.g., journal articles), while observational research codes personal interactions. This chapter will also describe outcome and process research. Outcome research evaluates whether treatments are effective, while process research helps us understand how change happens. Finally, we will look at the strengths and limitations of cross-sectional and longitudinal research, both of which are used to study changes over time.

A POTPOURRI OF RESEARCH DESIGNS

Meta-Analysis

Imagine that you want to know if premarital counseling is effective. How would you go about answering this question? One approach would be to locate and review all the experimental studies that have evaluated some form of premarital counseling. However, comparing results across all these studies might be difficult. The studies will include different approaches to premarital counseling, as well as different ways or instruments for measuring effectiveness. How might you derive a conclusion about the overall effectiveness of premarital counseling given these differences across studies?

The answer is **meta-analysis**, which can combine results across multiple studies in a particular area (Wampler, Reifman, & Serovich, 2005). Meta-analysis is able to accomplish this by calculating a statistic called an **effect size** for each experimental comparison. Because the effect size is a standardized score,[1] it allows us to compare or compile results across studies. Calculating an effect size takes all of our apples and oranges and coverts them into a common statistic—fruits. We can now calculate an average effect size across all the studies, which will allow us to examine the effectiveness of premarital counseling.

Typically meta-analyses are used to summarize results from multiple experimental studies where a particular treatment is compared to some other condition such as a no-treatment control or an alternative treatment. Effect sizes indicate how much better the treatment is compared to the comparison condition. Effect sizes close to zero mean the treatment is not any more effective than the comparison condition. A positive effect size means the treatment is more effective than the comparison condition, while a negative effect size means the comparison condition was more effective than the treatment. The greater the difference between the groups, the larger the effect size will be. Effect sizes based on the difference between groups (d statistic) are weak if they are 0.20, medium if they are 0.50, and large if they are 0.80 and above (Cohen, 1988). A meta-analysis by Carroll and Doherty (2003) found an average effect size of 0.80 when looking at seven experimental studies that compared a pre-

---

[1] When comparing two groups in an experimental study, the effect size (d) is typically calculated by dividing the difference between the groups by the combined (pooled) standard deviation of both groups. This results in a standardized score that is independent of the original unit of measure, thus making it possible to compare results across studies. Effect sizes can also be calculated from correlations.

marital counseling approach to a no-treatment control. Thus, premarital counseling appears to be quite effective.

Effect sizes can also be expressed in terms of what percentage of people are better off after receiving the treatment compared to those that do not. Based on the effect size ($d = 0.80$) for premarital counseling, Carroll and Doherty (2003) concluded "that this means that the average person who participated in a premarital prevention program was better off after the program than 79% of the people who did not receive a similar educational experience" (p. 113).

Effect sizes can also be calculated from correlations. Thus, meta-analyses can be used to combine results from nonexperimental research. For example, Jose, O'Leary, and Moyer (2010) wanted to know if premarital cohabitation was related to poorer marital outcomes. Using a meta-analysis of 16 studies, they discovered that individuals who had cohabitated were more likely to divorce than those who had never cohabitated. Effect sizes based on correlations (r statistic) are small at 0.10, medium at 0.30, and large if 0.50 and above (Cohen, 1988).

Meta-analysis has multiple advantages over the traditional method of reviewing the literature. First, meta-analysis can succinctly summarize the results of a large number of studies in terms of an effect size. It would be difficult to describe a large number of studies in a narrative form that is used in a traditional literature review. Second, meta-analysis allows one to quantify the magnitude of the treatment effect. This is more helpful than simply stating there is a statistically significant difference between the treatment and the comparison group. Third, meta-analysis can be more sensitive to detecting smaller treatment effects across multiple studies. Traditional literature reviews base their conclusions on whether studies show statistically significant results or not. However, this may underestimate the effectiveness of a treatment if sample sizes are small, which makes it more difficult to find statistically significant differences.

A fourth advantage of meta-analysis is that it can allow us to determine if certain factors influence the magnitude of the effect size. For example, do methodologically stronger studies have higher or lower effect sizes compared to weaker studies? Is the magnitude of the effect size dependent upon whether self-report or observational measures are used? It can also determine if the treatment is more successful for different types of outcomes. For example, Carroll and Doherty (2003) found the average effect size for premarital counseling was higher when comparing outcome measures that looked at communication processes compared to those that measured relationship quality. This is not a surprising result given that these programs often target improving communication, and most premarital couples already endorse high relationship satisfaction.

Recently researchers are adding **influence analyses** to meta-analysis to determine which studies have the most impact on the overall effect size (Baldwin, Christian, Berkeljon, Shadish, & Bean, 2012). It is possible, for example, that results from one or two studies with unusual results could inflate or deflate the overall effect size. An influence analysis allows one to identify these studies and determine their impact.

A critical issue in doing a meta-analysis is the selection of studies to be included in the study. For example, will the meta-analysis only include randomized controlled trials, or will quasi-experimental designs also be included? Researchers should also make explicit how they attempted to find all the relevant studies to make sure important studies are not overlooked or excluded. This often includes stating which databases were searched, and the keywords used to identify relevant studies.

A related issue is whether researchers should include unpublished studies (e.g., dissertations). Locating unpublished studies may be challenging and require more work. However, if they are not included, a potential publication bias could exist (Baldwin et al., 2012). Using only published studies raises the possibility that studies that did not find significant results will be underrepresented in the analysis because journals may be less likely to publish articles where there are no significant results. In addition, researchers may be less likely to submit these studies because they fear they will not be published.

Reversal (ABA and ABAB) and Multiple-Baseline Designs

The effectiveness of a treatment will sometimes be evaluated using reversal designs or a multiple-baseline design. These designs might be employed if there are a limited number of subjects. In **reversal designs**, the researcher evaluates the impact of administering and withdrawing the treatment to see if the treatment had an effect. The researcher first establishes a baseline (A) before administering the treatment. The treatment (B) is then administered to determine if it has a positive effect. The treatment is then withdrawn (A) to see if the problem returns to baseline. This is sometimes referred to an **ABA design**.

The withdrawal is necessary to give assurance that the change is due to the treatment and not some other factor. The following clinical example illustrates why the reversal can improve confidence with regard to internal validity.

Jefferson is a 6-year-old boy that is being seen by a family therapist intern for possible ADHD. His teacher requested that he be evaluated based on his behavior in the classroom (e.g., hyperactivity, impulsivity, inattention). The therapist concurs that Jefferson likely has ADHD, so she makes a referral for him to be seen by a psychiatrist for further evaluation and possible medication. The psychiatrist evaluates Jefferson in early June, and decides to prescribe medication for his ADHD. The mother is instructed to observe his behavior for 2 weeks to see if she notices any changes in his behavior. The mother notices that her son's behavior seems to have improved, which she attributes to the medication. However, the beginning of the medication trial corresponds with Jefferson finishing his school year. Could being out of school explain his change in behavior, particularly because he does not have the pressure of meeting expectations in a structured classroom? If Jefferson is taken off his medication and he goes back to his earlier problematic behaviors, then this will provide greater confidence that the medication was indeed working, and was simply not an artifact of him being out of school.

If you subsequently administer the treatment again (B) and measure its impact, then you have an **ABAB design**. If reintroducing the treatment creates another positive change (e.g., Jefferson's behavior improves once he is put back on the medication again), then you have even more confidence that the effect is due to treatment and not some other factor.

Reversal designs work best if the treatment results in a clear and immediate effect. For example, it would be difficult to test antidepressants using this design since the benefit may not be evident until 4 to 6 weeks after treatment begins. In addition, the effects of the treatment must disappear after the treatment is withdrawn. Many interventions do not work in this way. For most interventions, we hope a permanent rather than temporary change has been introduced.

The **multiple-baseline design** is an alternative to the reversal designs that circumvents this last problem. A baseline is measured for each individual in the study. The treatment is staggered across individuals so no one receives the treatment at the same time (see Figure 7.1). If each person improves after receiving the treatment, then the change is likely due to the treatment rather than outside factors that would likely impact study participants simultaneously.

Content Analysis

Content analysis studies the content of some form of recorded media or communication, such as TV shows, movies, speeches, or publications. In

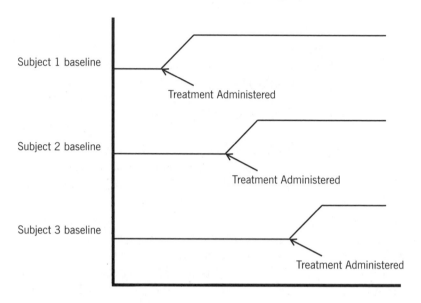

FIGURE 7.1. Example of multiple-baseline design. In this example, the treatment appears to be effective, given that there is a change in the baseline for each subject after the treatment is introduced.

family therapy, content analysis often examines the content of journal articles to see what trends are evident in the field. For example, three studies (Flori, 1989; Lambert-Shute & Fruhauf, 2011; Van Amburg, Barber, & Zimmerman, 1996) have explored over time the extent to which later life issues have been addressed in the family therapy literature. Results from all three studies indicate that limited attention has been given to later life issues.

When doing a content analysis, researchers first define the overall purpose of the study and the specific research questions they hope to answer. Lambert-Shute and Fruhauf (2011) wanted to explore how family therapy literature between 1997 and 2006 addressed later life issues. They also had more specific research questions they wanted to answer, such as "What types of presenting problems are mentioned in connection with older adults?" and "What types of family therapy theories are represented in the articles with a focus on later life family concerns?" (p. 29).

Researchers then develop **coding systems** to answer each research question. A coding system has predetermined categories developed by the researcher for recording data. For example, Lambert-Shute and Fruhauf (2011) coded articles as to whether or not they had a focus on later life issues. For articles that had a later life focus, they had additional coding systems to evaluate what presenting problems or theories were mentioned in relationship to working with older adults.

Researchers need to evaluate if the coding system has good interrater reliability to ensure there is consistency or agreement on how things are coded across raters (see Chapter 2). Lambert-Shute and Fruhauf independently coded each of the articles, and then compared their results. They reported a 92% or higher agreement for all coding categories.

An important part of a content analysis is defining what materials will be studied. Lambert-Shute and Fruhauf (2011) decided to examine articles published in three leading family therapy journals: *Journal of Marital and Family Therapy*, *American Journal of Family Therapy*, and *Contemporary Family Therapy*. They examined all 957 articles published in these journals for a 10-year period. In some cases, researchers may select a sample of articles (e.g., every fifth article) from a larger population of articles.

One potential limitation of a content analysis is that it may not perfectly reflect what is happening in a field. For example, aging issues could potentially be receiving greater attention in training programs than is reflected in the published literature. Content analyses may also miss emerging trends due to the possible significant delay between data collection and the eventual publication of the results. For example, the Lambert-Shute and Fruhauf study was published in 2011, but the articles studied were only up to 2006. Nonetheless, content analyses can provide important insights into how much attention certain topics or issues have received within the field.

Observational Research

Observational research (also known as **systematic observation**) is the careful measurement and recording of specific behaviors in a specified setting. This approach is different from the naturalistic observation that is done in a qualitative ethnography (Chapter 6) because it focuses on a narrower range of behaviors. It also uses a coding system to measure behaviors rather than using a narrative to describe them. Table 7.1 shows an example of a simple coding system that can be used to measure therapist behavior during a session.

**TABLE 7.1. Example of a Coding System:
Therapist Resistance Code**

1. *Support*—Positive responses toward the client that show warmth, humor, understanding, or encouragement.

2. *Teach*—Providing information about parenting, family-life, or other therapy-related issues; responses that serve to structure or manage the session.

3. *Question*—Responses that seek information.

4. *Confront*—Responses that tend to challenge the client, including disagreement, disapproval, and negative, sarcastic, or hostile comments.

5. *Reframe*—Reconstructions of what another person has said, such that the result is something different from the way it was initially stated.

6. *Talk*—Response cannot be coded with another category, including unintelligible verbalizations, conversations about the weather, scheduling, etc.

7. *Facilitate*—Responses primarily indicating the therapist is listening to the client, such as "um-humm," "yeah," "right," or "sure."

Note. Based on Forgatch and Chamberlain (1982).

For a coding system to be effective, it must possess several qualities. First, the categories must be exhaustive. In other words, it must include all the possible behaviors that might be observed in the setting. Second, the categories must be mutually exclusive. This is to ensure that raters using the coding system are not confused as to which category a behavior belongs. Third, categories must be clearly defined so that raters can easily identify in which category a behavior belongs.

Similar to what we discussed with content analysis, coding systems in observational research are evaluated for interrater reliability. There needs to be consistency or close agreement between raters on how they categorize behaviors using the coding system. Interrater reliabilities should ideally be .80 and above. Interrater reliabilities for each category may be reported, and may be less than .80 in some cases. There should also be evidence for the validity of the coding system. Scores from a coding scale can be correlated with other measures of similar or different constructs to establish criterion or construct validity (see Chapter 2 for a more detailed discussion of measurement validity).

If they are simple enough, coding systems can be used in real time to record observed behavior. In most cases, however, coding interactions is more complicated. Typically, what is being observed (e.g., a therapy session) is videotaped and subsequently coded. This allows individuals to stop and start the video to record behaviors. Due to the time-consuming nature of this process, researchers often use students as coders. To ensure they are using the coding system properly, coders must be carefully trained.

Observational research is a quantitative approach to collecting data. Behaviors can be quantified into numbers using a coding system, generating scores that can be used in statistical analyses. For example, one study (Robbins, Liddle, Turner, Dakof, Alexander, & Kogan, 2006) used an observational coding system to measure the strength of the therapeutic alliance between the therapist and family members seeking help for a drug-abusing adolescent. They found the therapeutic alliance significantly declined from the first to the second session for families that later dropped out of treatment, but it remained the same for those that completed treatment. This supports the importance of attending to the therapeutic relationship, especially in the early stages of therapy.

Observational research can be used to measure key variables in other study designs such as experiments. For example, observational rating scales were used to measure couple communication patterns in a study that compared integrative behavioral couple therapy to traditional behavioral couple therapy (Baucom, Sevier, Eldridge, Doss, & Christensen, 2011).

Outcome Research

The goal of **outcome research** is to determine if a treatment is effective, or how its effectiveness may compare to an alternative treatment. Outcome research is typically done using experimental designs discussed in Chapter 3. However, reversal (ABA, ABAB) and multiple-baseline designs can also be used to test treatment effectiveness.

When designing outcome research, the researcher must take into consideration multiple factors on how to evaluate the effectiveness of a treatment. Many of these considerations are interrelated. First, the researcher must decide whether a successful outcome is based on resolving the presenting issue or a change of family dynamics. Although we would anticipate both would occur concurrently, it is possible that we may have one but not the other.

Second, should we base our treatment effectiveness on client self-report or observed behavioral change? Many researchers prefer measuring change using observational research because it is often less reactive than using self-report measures. However, focusing exclusively on behavioral changes overlooks assessing client satisfaction, which some consider to be an important outcome measure. In addition, observational research will be unable to assess the meaning that clients attach to what is happening in their lives. In some cases, a shift in perspective may be the most important change that happens in therapy.

Third, the researcher must decide whether outcome measures will focus on the individual or the relationship. Measuring individuals is much easier, and will permit you to assess client satisfaction and changes in each individual's thoughts, feelings, and behaviors (which may differ among family members). However, the goal of many family therapists is to change the relationship dynamics as a way to resolve presenting problems. From this perspective, the relationship rather than the individual would need to be measured.

However, measuring a relationship is complicated and requires more than simply averaging the scores of all family members. Let us use two couples to illustrate this point. On the Dyadic Adjustment Scale, Amanda and Joshua both score 90, which is in the mildly distressed range. In comparison, Alicia scores a 60 and Fernando scores a 120. Thus, Alicia is severely distressed, while Fernando seems quite happy in the relationship. Although both couples would have an average score of 90, it is quite apparent that the scores do not represent how different the couples are qualitatively. Thus, it can be a challenge for the researcher to find a way to accurately measure a relationship.

The above discussion implies that the decisions around measuring outcomes will be either/or propositions. In reality, researchers may choose to take a both/and approach. For example, they may try to assess both the extent to which the presenting issue has been resolved (e.g., reduced drug use by an adolescent) and if there is a change in family dynamics. Likewise, a researcher may include both observational research and self-report measures to measure multiple outcome variables. Stronger studies will look at outcomes from a number of different perspectives.

The amount of change is just one criterion upon which a treatment's effectiveness can be evaluated. Gurman and Kniskern (1981) suggest several factors that can be considered when comparing the effectiveness of two treatments. Can one treatment be done more briefly than the other? Also, can one treatment be done more economically than another? Obviously a briefer form of treatment will be more cost effective than a treatment that requires more sessions to be equally effective. A treatment that can be effectively delivered through group therapy will also be more economical than one that cannot. In addition, a treatment that can be administered by paraprofessionals will also be more cost effective than one that requires licensed mental health providers.

You can also evaluate if one treatment leads to a higher dropout rate. This problem could arise if one treatment is psychologically more difficult to do. For example, a treatment for PTSD that requires extensive exposure to previous trauma may be more difficult for a client to do than one that does not require the same level of exposure.

Finally, the long-term impact of treatment should be considered. Is one treatment better at clients maintaining their treatment gains over time? Has the effectiveness of one treatment been documented for a longer period of time than another?

Process Research

Another type of psychotherapy research is **process research**. As the name implies, this type of research is focused on the processes that occur in therapy. Whereas outcome research examines if there has been change, process research is concerned with how the change occurred. Process research often accomplishes this by looking at critical events that occur in therapy, and then measuring if there was a positive outcome for this event.

Process research has evolved over time. Process research has traditionally focused on studying how change occurs in therapy by using the observational research methods described earlier. Thus, therapy sessions are videotaped and interactions analyzed using coding systems. However, process researchers also recognize the need to understand the thoughts and emotions that clients and therapists experience in therapy. Therefore, some researchers have used self-report instruments to collect this information. The best process research often collects both types of data (Lebow, 2006).

Some researchers have employed a discovery-oriented approach to studying therapy called **task analysis** (Bradley & Johnson, 2005). Using this approach, researchers study critical events in therapy and try to uncover patterns that lead to either successful or unsuccessful outcomes. For example, Bradley and Furrow (2004) studied several taped sessions of therapists who successfully created softening events in couples therapy, which is an important intervention in emotionally focused therapy. Using task analysis, the researchers were able to articulate the steps therapists took to create softening events.

Process research can aid in the development of **micro-theories** that can guide therapists in their moment-to-moment decisions in therapy. Family therapy theories such as structural family therapy help point us to where we want to go (e.g., strengthen boundaries, strengthen the hierarchy), but they do not give us the step-by-step directions on how to get there. The hope is that micro-theories developed through process research can do this.

Cross-Sectional and Longitudinal Research

Human beings change over time. This is most evident when we study children and adolescents. However, adults also change and mature over time. Couples and families also go through changes as they move through the family life cycle. Thus, researchers may be interested in studying how individuals or relationships change over time.

Cross-sectional research and longitudinal research are two approaches to studying how things change over time. In **cross-sectional research**, individuals (or relationships) of different ages are studied at the same time. For example, a researcher might collect data from a group of 3-year-old children, and compare it to a group of 6-year-old children measured at the same time to see how they are different. In contrast, **longitudinal research** would collect data from the group of 3-year-old children, and then measure the same group again when they turn six to see how they changed.

Both approaches have strengths and limitations. Obviously, cross-sectional research takes less time to complete. In the above example, one does not need to wait 3 years to finish collecting the data using the longitudinal design. The longer the longitudinal study lasts, the more problems that can arise. For example, you may lose contact with participants or they may drop out of the study. There is also a risk that a longitudinal study may lose its funding. In some cases, the research questions may become trivial or obsolete as new information from other studies emerges over time.

However, cross-sectional research can suffer from issues with internal validity that can arise from **cohort effects**. With cross-sectional research, if we find differences between the groups, it is possible they are due to each group (or cohort) having a different history. For example, if we were interested in knowing if individuals change their views on gender roles over time, we could compare a group of 20-year-old individuals to a group of 70-year-old individuals to see if there was a difference. If we found that 70-year-old individuals had more traditional views on gender roles than 20-year-olds, could we safely conclude that individuals become more traditional in their views of gender over time? Due to possible cohort effects, the answer is no. It is possible that the difference reflects the fact that the 70-year-old individuals were born and raised before the women's movement, whereas the 20-year-old individuals were born after it. This could account for the difference rather than changes over time being due to aging. With longitudinal research, there are no concerns with cohort effects because the same group is followed over time.

APPLICATION

Evaluating Meta-analyses

There are a number of questions you can ask when evaluating the quality of a meta-analysis. First, you should look at the studies included in the analysis. The researcher should clearly specify what types of studies were eligible for inclusion. Do you agree with the criteria used, or do you feel they excluded important studies? Also, did they include both published and unpublished studies? If unpublished studies were not included, then be aware that a publication bias may exist. Do you believe the researcher did a good job searching for all the relevant studies based on the databases and keywords used? Finally, how many studies were available for the meta-analysis? Generally, stronger conclusions can be drawn from areas where there are more studies.

Second, you should evaluate how the analysis was done. The researcher should be transparent in describing the decisions made in conducting the analysis, such as being explicit in stating how the effect size was calculated because there are variations in how to do this. Stronger studies will rate the methodological quality of studies used in the analysis, and then determine if this rating is related to effect size. Stronger studies will also examine if other factors (e.g., type of outcome measures, sample size, client characteristics) are related to effect sizes. More recent meta-analyses may also include an influence analysis to determine if certain studies significantly impact the effect size more than others, which enhances the rigor of the study.

Third, what clinical implications can be drawn from the study? It is important to be clear on what the comparison group is upon which the effect size is based. Was the treatment compared to a no treatment, an alternative treatment, or treatment as usual? If the latter, then it can be helpful to know what treatment as usual looks like for that presenting problem. You should also consider the magnitude of the effect size. This will help you gauge the practical significance of the results. For effect sizes based on differences (d), 0.20 is small, 0.50 is medium, and 0.80 and above is large. For effect sizes based on correlations (r), then 0.10 is small, 0.30 is medium, and 0.50 and above is large.

Reversal (ABA and ABAB) and Multiple–Baseline Designs

Some of the considerations for evaluating reversal and multiple-baseline designs are similar to those discussed with experiments. Were the treatments clearly described? Also, is there evidence the treatments were delivered as intended?

Are there any concerns with internal validity? For reversal designs, you will have more confidence that the change can be attributed to the treatment with an ABAB design compared to an ABA design. For both reversal and multiple-baseline designs, confidence in internal validity increases if treatment leads to an immediate and pronounced effect rather than one which is small and gradual. Sample size can also impact confidence in internal validity, particularly for multiple-baseline designs. The more individuals who have a corresponding improvement after receiving the treatment, the more confidence you can have in attributing the change to the treatment.

Due to the very small sizes, questions of external validity naturally arise. Establishing external validity using these designs is similar to qualitative research. The researcher should provide a clear description of the subjects so the reader can compare them to the individuals (e.g., clients) with whom he or she would like to apply the findings. If the two groups are similar, then the likelihood the findings will generalize increases.

You may recognize that we use the logic of the multiple-baseline design to evaluate our interventions in clinical practice. For example, you might instruct a depressed client to record her automatic thoughts and challenge any cognitive distortions. If your client reports a reduction in depressive symptoms upon her return to therapy the following week, you may conclude that your intervention worked. However, it is possible that it is simply a coincidence. Perhaps your client received a new job offer or raise, which improved her mood. If you prescribe the same intervention to another depressed client and get a similar positive result, then you have more faith that the intervention works. With each new client that you successfully treat using this intervention, your confidence in its effectiveness increases.

Content Analysis

There are a number of factors to consider when evaluating a content analysis. First, you should evaluate the coding system. Did the researcher clearly describe how the materials were analyzed and coded? Did the researcher provide any evidence for the interrater reliability of the coding system?

Second, evaluate the appropriateness of the materials (e.g., journal articles) included in the study. If a researcher did a content analysis of journal articles, do you agree with the researcher's decisions regarding what journals to include? Do you have any concerns about how representative these journals are? Did the researcher include all the articles within the stated time frame, or was a portion sampled? If sampling was done, was this done in an appropriate fashion?

Third, did the researcher draw appropriate conclusions from the study based on the content that was analyzed? Issues of external validity are important here. The ability to generalize from the study will depend upon how representative the articles or media are. For example, a content analysis of journals with a strong research focus may not reflect what might be found in journals with a strong practitioner focus. As discussed earlier, it is also important that the research not overstate the extent to which the findings represent the field as a whole. Journal articles may not always perfectly mirror what happens in practice within a field.

Evaluating Observational Research

Obviously one of the most important considerations in evaluating observational research is the quality of the coding system. If the researcher describes the coding system, do the categories appear to be exhaustive, mutually exclusive, and clearly defined? The researcher should report interrater reliability for the coding system, which ideally should be .80 and above. The researcher will often report the range of reliabilities for each category. It is not unusual for some specific codes or categories to be below .80. In addition to interrater reliability, there should also be some evidence for the validity of the coding system. If the researcher is using a preexisting coding system, he or she may simply refer the reader to the original research.

Stronger studies will also discuss who did the coding, and what steps were taken to ensure the coding was done properly. This is often accomplished by training the raters until their ratings closely match those of the researcher when coding something.

When observational research is used as the primary design (rather than an element of the design), you evaluate it like you would other quantitative designs. Is the purpose clearly defined, and has the researcher stated the specific questions being studied? Are there concerns about external validity (see Chapter 4) based on the sample that was used? Results may not generalize if the sample is unique in some way. You should also be attentive to issues relating to internal validity. If results are correlational, some of the concerns we noted in Chapter 3 (e.g., direction of cause and effect, spurious relationships) may impact internal validity. Good researchers will clearly articulate the limitations of the study for the reader.

Outcome Research

Evaluating outcome research begs the question "How do you measure success in therapy?" This is an important question for both researchers and clinicians. If Suzanne tells you that she thinks therapy has helped her, but it does not appear that she has made significant changes in how she lives her life, can we trust her report that therapy has been a success? Or, should we expect that there should be some behavioral changes to reflect real change? Some researchers might argue that we cannot trust self-report measures because they are vulnerable to social desirability and demand characteristics, and that measuring change should ideally be based on observable changes in behavior. Thus, some might not view Suzanne's therapy as a success. However, others might argue that a change in perception can be as important as a change in behavior. For example, some therapies like integrative behavioral couples therapy incorporate the concept of acceptance, which requires a change in perception rather than a change in behavior.

Perhaps the key to assessing effectiveness of therapy, whether it is research or our own work, is to evaluate it from multiple perspectives. Although self-report measures like satisfaction are subject to reactivity (e.g., social desirability and demand characteristics), they are also the best approach for assessing if there has been a change of perception. However, there is also value in assessing if someone other than the client (e.g., therapist, researcher) can observe a change either in the individual's behavior or relationship dynamics. Both perspectives can be valuable. Indeed, the more indicators we use to assess change, the more confidence we can have in determining if therapy has been successful. We will be more assured that our therapy was successful if the client reports feeling better (self-report) and if we also observe behavioral changes by the client. Furthermore, if the client reports that others have commented on the changes they have witnessed, this gives us even greater confidence.

In a similar manner, stronger outcome studies will evaluate effectiveness from multiple angles. Rather than rely just on self-report or observational measures, they will include both. They may not only assess whether there has been a reduction in the presenting problem, but they will attempt to measure if there has been a change in couple or family dynamics.

Process Research

Therapists may find process research particularly valuable in their clinical work. As we discussed earlier, process research is working toward developing micro-theories for how to create change. In the area of emotionally focused therapy, process research has identified the steps to creating softening events (Bradley & Furrow, 2004), or how to work through attachment injuries (Makinen & Johnson, 2006). This kind of information can be invaluable in providing therapists with a road map for creating change.

We discussed task analysis as one approach for doing process research. Through taping and studying their own sessions, therapists can examine critical events in their therapy sessions to determine what factors led to a successful or unsuccessful outcome. If a therapist is systematic in choosing a certain type of critical event to study across sessions, he or she might be able to uncover steps that could be followed with future clients to successfully create change.

Cross-sectional and Longitudinal Research

When a cross-sectional study is done, one must consider the possibility of cohort effects. Has the researcher identified this as a limitation and what possible cohorts effects might need to be considered? For longitudinal research, a key threat is losing individuals over time, either because they cannot be located or they refuse to continue to participate. This can have implications if the individuals who drop out are different from those that remain in the study. The researcher should discuss how many have dropped out of the study over time, and describe efforts to determine how they may be different from those who continue to be followed.

CHAPTER 8

Ethics and Values in Research

In a well-publicized case, nearly 400 black men with syphilis were observed beginning in 1932 for over 40 years to study the course of the illness. Known as the Tuskegee study, the research gained notoriety due to the ethical concerns surrounding it. A panel that reviewed the study found the men were not given sufficient information about the study or its purpose. Amazingly, the infected men were never offered penicillin many years later when it became known as an effective treatment for syphilis. A class action lawsuit was eventually filed against the United States government, which resulted in a large out-of-court settlement (Centers for Disease Control and Prevention, 2011). This study is a tragic example of how the researchers' duty to avoid causing harm to participants was ignored.

Researchers are expected to follow several principles to minimize the risk of harming research participants. They must first demonstrate that the benefits of the study outweigh the costs. The potential benefits and costs of participating in a study should also be provided before individuals agree to be in a study to ensure informed consent. Participation also needs to be voluntary. Researchers should also strive to protect the privacy of participants through various means, such as offering confidentiality or anonymity. As an additional safeguard, ethics committees (e.g., institutional review boards) within universities or organizations review proposed research to ensure it will be conducted in a safe manner. We will explore each of these principles in greater depth in this chapter, along with the potential for dishonesty in research.

We will also discuss the role of values in research. Specifically, we will examine whether it is possible for researchers to truly separate themselves from what they are studying, thereby making their inquiry value-free. We will also explore how some researchers (e.g., feminist researchers) believe our values should guide our research to bring about positive change in society.

ETHICAL CONSIDERATIONS IN RESEARCH

Potential for Harm

Researchers must carefully consider the potential for physical or psychological harm that individuals may experience if they participate in a study. Research that provokes strong emotions such as anger or fear may signal possible psychological harm. Emotional harm can also arise by creating significant stress, damaging a person's self-esteem, or encouraging an individual to perform illegal or immoral acts. In a highly controversial study conducted by a researcher named Milgram (1963), research participants were instructed to administer electrical shocks to another person whenever they incorrectly answered a question. Milgram wanted to determine how far individuals would go in following an authority figure, even to the point of causing serious harm to another individual. Milgram wanted to study this phenomenon because many of the individuals who committed Nazi atrocities during World War II claimed they were only following orders. In Milgram's study, many of the participants followed the researcher's instructions by administering increasingly higher levels of shock to the point of causing harm, potentially even death. Participants experienced significant emotional distress while they were giving the shocks. In reality, the individuals receiving the electrical shocks were actually research assistants, and only pretended to be hurt by the shocks while hidden behind a wall from the participants.

Researchers must consider a number of factors when assessing the potential for harm. First, they must try to anticipate what types of harm may occur. For example, a study asking individuals about their past child abuse may recreate negative feelings from the past, such as sadness or anger. Second, they must estimate the likelihood harm will occur. Are individuals likely to experience a potential for harm, or is the chance of it happening small? Third, what will be the impact if harm should occur? Will it be mild or severe? Will it be long-lasting or temporary? If harm occurs, is it reversible? It may be acceptable to expose a research participant to a stressful situation provided the level of stress is mild and brief because the risk of permanent psychological harm is minimal.

If there is a potential for harm, researchers need to take certain precautions. For example, researchers may debrief individuals at the conclusion of a study to be certain participation did not cause emotional harm. This is especially important if the study used deception. In the Milgram study, participants were debriefed after the study to reassure them no one had actually been harmed. Another precaution is to exclude individuals who are at most risk for experiencing harm. Studies that treat depressed individuals may exclude those who express any suicidal ideation. Decisions like this may be justified on ethical grounds, but may impact the external validity of the findings.

Principles That Guide Ethical Research

There are a number of principles researchers follow to ensure their work is done in a safe manner. The first principle is that the benefits of the study must outweigh its costs. It is incumbent on the researcher to make a case as to the benefits of doing the study. Determining if the benefits outweigh the costs may be difficult at times because it may be hard to know what the benefits or costs will be. In addition, the benefits and costs may be hard to quantify, making it difficult to accurately weigh the ratio of benefits to costs. Due to the fact that weighing of the cost–benefit ratio can be subjective, it is important that someone other than the researcher reviews the study because a potential conflict of interest may bias the researcher's assessment. Finally, one must consider who will receive the benefits and who will incur the costs. Many studies provide a benefit by adding to our body of knowledge, but do not directly benefit the study participants.

The second principle is that participation in research should be voluntary. Individuals should not be coerced or pressured to be in a study. One way this can happen is if the researcher has a dual relationship with those being recruited for the study, creating the possibility for negative consequences to arise if the individuals do not participate. For example, students may agree to be in a study conducted by their professor if they fear their grade could be impacted if they do not. In another example, a military officer wanted to conduct his dissertation with those under his command. It is unlikely that individuals in his command would have felt participation was truly voluntary had he been given permission to conduct the study. Offering a large incentive for being in a study can also compromise the voluntary nature of a study by making it difficult to decline participation. This is especially a concern when recruiting individuals from a vulnerable population. For example, individuals who are poor may feel compelled to participate in a study if it offers a large monetary incentive, even if there are significant risks.

Protecting privacy is the third principle required for conducting ethical research. There are a number of safeguards researchers can follow to protect privacy, including offering confidentiality or anonymity. **Confidentiality** means the researcher knows who the participants are, but will not disclose their identities to anyone outside the study. **Anonymity** is different from confidentiality in that even the researcher does not know the research participants' identities, which provides greater protection than confidentiality. Another safeguard that can be used in quantitative studies is the reporting of **aggregate data**, which combines individual responses and reports only summary statistics such as percentages, averages, or median scores. Aggregating the data makes it impossible to know how any one individual responded, thus protecting each person's privacy.

Qualitative studies present unique challenges for protecting privacy because individual responses (e.g., quotes) are often reported. In addition, the qualitative researcher may describe the setting and participants in sufficient detail so that it may be possible to guess the identity of one or more individuals. To minimize this possibility, qualitative researchers use pseudonyms. However, this may not be a sufficient safeguard, particularly if some of the participants hold a visible position within the setting or have some other unique characteristics. For example, if a study described the experience of therapists in a training program, it may be possible to attribute a quote to a particular person if the individual possesses unique characteristics such as race/ethnicity, age, or gender. If the study included faculty perspectives, quotes by the program director would allow one to identify the individual's identity if the program could be guessed or is known. In qualitative studies, individuals should be told what steps will be used to protect privacy, but warned that it may not be possible to guarantee confidentiality. If they are concerned about their privacy, they can elect not to participate, or carefully consider their remarks based on the knowledge that others may be able to later identify them.

Obtaining **informed consent** is the fourth principle. Prior to participating in a study, individuals should be told important information about the study, such as the purpose, potential benefits or risks from participating, and how their privacy will be protected. Based on this information, individuals can then decide whether it is appropriate for them to participate in the study. In the case of minors or adults whose judgment is impaired (e.g., Alzheimer's, intellectual disabilities), adults responsible for their care are also required to consent to the study.

In some cases, effectively studying a phenomenon may require some deception. Otherwise, telling individuals the purpose of the study will alter their behavior. For example, if participants in the Milgram study knew the true purpose of the study, it is likely they would have changed how they behaved. However, using deception makes it impossible to have fully informed consent. If deception is used, then the risk of harm must be low. Researchers should also debrief individuals afterwards to reveal the true purpose of the study and to ensure no harm has occurred.

Another principle researchers follow is to have peers review their study for potential ethical issues. Universities and other organizations typically have a committee, often called an institutional review board, which is devoted to reviewing research studies for ethical concerns. Researchers in these organizations must obtain approval from the review board or committee before they can conduct the study.

Dishonesty in Research

Although uncommon, dishonesty in research can and does exist. Dishonesty can happen in different ways. In some cases, a researcher may alter or create fictional data. A Dutch psychologist by the name of Diederik Stapel was recently discovered to have manipulated or even fabricated data in at least 30 peer-reviewed journal articles (Callaway, 2011).

Another form of dishonesty is to only publish data that supports a researcher's hypotheses and withhold findings that contradict them. For example, Smith (2005) has noted that some pharmaceutical companies will selectively publish findings that support the efficacy of their drugs. This can lead to an inflated sense of the efficacy of a drug or intervention. One study compared all of the results reported to the U.S. Food and Drug Administration (FDA) for 12 antidepressants to the subset of results that were actually published (Turner, Matthews, Linardatos, Tell, & Rosenthal, 2008). The results for the published studies were more positive than those that were not published, although it was not possible to determine if the other studies were not submitted for publication or if they were not accepted for publication (or both). Using meta-analysis, the authors found the effect size associated with the antidepressants was 32% larger on the basis of the published studies alone.

When reviewing studies, it is important to be aware of potential conflicts of interest that may impact the research. Bekelman, Li, and Gross (2003) reviewed several studies in biomedical research that examined the potential role of conflict of interest on study findings. They found a significant relationship between industry sponsorship of a study and results being favorable to the industry.

VALUES IN RESEARCH

Researchers take different positions on the role of values in research. Our discussion of values in research will center on two important questions. Can research be value-free, and secondly, should research be value-free?

Researchers have debated the first question of whether research can be value-free. Some researchers believe there is an objective reality that can be known independent of the observer. In other words, who the researcher is, including his or her values, can be separated from what is being studied. Researchers who take this stance have been called positivists. However, many researchers believe it is not possible to separate the observer from what is being studied. What we see and know is shaped by who we are, including our values. These researchers go by a variety of names, including post-positivists, postmodernists, or constructivists.

As a general rule, qualitative researchers believe that reality is socially constructed. What we understand "reality" to be is shaped by who we are and the social context in which we are embedded. Therefore, qualitative researchers would disagree with the positivist position that we are separate from what we are studying. That is why qualitative researchers describe themselves so that the reader can understand how the researcher's background may influence the collection and interpretation of the data.

Although quantitative researchers can be either positivists or post-positivists, they seldom include a description of themselves in their studies. This practice seems to imply that it is not necessary to know the researcher's qualities because they do not influence the study. This is consistent with the positivist view that who the researcher is and what is being studied can be independent of one another. However, a post-positivist would state that the researcher's values and background have the potential to influence the collection and interpretation of data whether the study is qualitative or quantitative in design.

The second question that researchers can differ upon is whether research should be value-free. Some researchers believe we should attempt to keep our values out of the process as much as possible to retain objectivity. Their goal is to understand how things are. Other researchers believe our values should inform our work. They would argue that simply studying things the way they are perpetuates the status quo, which at times may be oppressive. They believe research should be used to promote social change.

Feminist research, for example, tries to create change in areas where oppression or inequalities may exist. Early feminist research focused on women's lack of power in society and families. Feminist researchers have expanded their research to include other disempowered or marginalized groups, such as children of abuse and minorities.

Feminist researchers have used a variety of methodological designs. One approach commonly used in feminist research is qualitative research. For example, Allen and Piercy (2005) have argued that autoethnography is a good fit with feminist inquiry because it can depict the experiences of a marginalized group using the researcher's own reflective account of their personal life. Consistent with qualitative research, feminists believe the role that the researcher's values and background have in the inquiry process needs to be acknowledged.

APPLICATION

Evaluating Ethical Considerations in Research

It may be difficult to assess if a study followed the ethical principles described in this chapter. It is often assumed that ethical procedures (e.g., obtaining informed consent, voluntary participation, peer review) were followed, although the reader is seldom told this directly. Some research articles, however, will include a statement that the study was evaluated and approved by the institution's review board. In addition, some studies may discuss a particular ethical issue, especially if it impacted the methods or design. For example, if deception was used, the study should discuss why this was necessary and how this was handled ethically.

Even if the researcher does not make explicit how ethical issues were addressed, you may be able to make some indirect assessment. The researcher should have made an argument in the literature review as to why the study is important, which helps you assess if the benefits outweigh the costs. Steps to protect privacy (e.g., offering confidentiality) may not be made explicit unless special safeguards were taken, such as offering anonymity because of the sensitive nature of the topic. You should also consider if a potential dual relationship exists between the researcher and the participants, which may compromise individuals' perceptions that participation was completely voluntary or their willingness to disclose sensitive information. Qualitative studies are most likely to make explicit the researcher's role or relationship with participants and its potential impact on the study.

Dishonesty in research may be difficult to evaluate. Increasingly, journals (especially in the medical field) are asking authors to disclose any potential conflicts of interest that may exist. For example, a researcher would need to disclose that they are being paid by a pharmaceutical company to evaluate an investigational drug. Be aware that a conflict of interest (e.g., sponsored research, evaluating one's own intervention) may be more likely to produce favorable results. Greater confidence can be placed on findings that have been replicated in other studies, especially those conducted by researchers who have not been involved in the development of the intervention or treatment.

Ethical Parallels with Clinical Work

Ethical issues in clinical work and research parallel each other. Neither therapy nor research should be conducted unless it is anticipated there will be a benefit. Both the researcher and the therapist should take steps to minimize harm, such as protecting privacy (e.g., confidentiality) and using informed consent. Peer review can be an important safeguard in both research and clinical work. In therapy, peer review typically takes the form of consulting with colleagues or seeking supervision. Finally, both the researcher and the clinician need to consider how dual relationships and conflicts of interest can create ethical problems.

Values in Research and Therapy

Most therapists, if asked to think about it, would probably align more with post-positivists than positivists. We frequently encounter clients whose belief about what the truth is may differ from other family members. Therefore, we recognize that what we perceive to be true is often dependent upon our frame of reference, which is consistent with a post-positivist view. If you are a post-positivist, then you should be asking yourself when evaluating research if the researcher's values, background, theoretical orientation, or other factors may influence the collection and interpretation of the data. Qualitative researchers are more likely to discuss this issue than quantitative researchers, although both should make explicit how theory has informed their research. Qualitative researchers are more likely to consider how other factors such as their values or background influence the study. However, similar forces may be at play in quantitative research even if the author does not explicitly acknowledge them.

We should also consider to what extent the researcher's values have deliberately shaped the study. For example, feminist researchers will often try to create change through their research. Do you agree with the researcher's aims? Has the researcher's goal of creating change through the research compromised the researcher's ability to be objective in the methodology used or interpretation of the data (as much as possible within a post-positivist framework)?

The same questions we posed about the role of values in research can also be asked about therapy. Most of us would probably agree that it is not possible for therapists to be completely value-free in how they do therapy. Our background, experiences, and values will shape our clinical work. In addition, most of us would probably conclude that therapy should not be completely value-free. For example, like researchers, we hold the value that no one should be harmed. Therefore, we will actively work to keep others safe if there is abuse or the threat of harm to self or others in therapy.

However, both researchers and therapists may struggle with how far to go in promoting their values. Some therapists will view traditional gender roles in therapy as perpetuating the inequality between men and women and will want to challenge them. Others may view traditional gender roles as a legitimate option for couples, and would not challenge a couple's choice if that is their desire. Therefore, where we draw the line in promoting our values is something with which both researchers and clinicians must grapple.

CHAPTER 9

Descriptive Statistics

$\mathbf{Y}$ou are sitting in class anxiously awaiting the results of your exam. Before passing the exam back to students, the instructor displays to the class the distribution of test scores. The instructor also reports that the class mean or average was a 79. You notice the distribution of scores appears to be somewhat bell-shaped, with the middle of the bell centered near the mean of 79. You also observe the majority of scores fall between 65 and 95. However, you notice one person did poorly on the exam, receiving a 45. You are hoping this is not your score!

If this situation seems familiar to you (as it should be with most students), then you are already familiar with the key concepts in this chapter. When we measure a variable, such as student knowledge of a particular topic, there is typically a variation in scores across individuals. A frequency distribution shows us how often certain values (e.g., test scores) are observed when measuring a variable across a particular group. Frequency distributions can be depicted pictorially using a bar graph or a histogram. Alternatively, how many times each response was given can be summarized in a frequency table.

Descriptive statistics can also be used to summarize the data, helping us convert large amounts of data into a manageable form. The mean or average exam score that the instructor provided is an example of a descriptive statistic. The mean, along with the median and mode, are measures of central tendency, which shows where the majority of scores tend to cluster. Descriptive statistics such as the range, standard deviation, and variance are used to represent how much spread or variation there is in the data.

We will also learn that the shape of a frequency distribution is important to researchers. Many phenomena follow a bell-shaped curve when mapped out, much like the exam scores in our example. Researchers call this a normal distribution. However, some distributions are skewed, with a greater number of scores on one side. Distributions can have extreme scores called outliers. The individual who did considerably poorer on the exam compared to the other students is an example of an outlier. Conversely, students who "ruin the curve" on an exam by vastly outperforming other students are also outliers.

THE BASICS OF DESCRIPTIVE STATISTICS

Describing Frequency Distributions

Imagine that you have collected information from 400 individuals on their marital satisfaction. Each person was asked to rate how happy they were in their marriage, using the following categories: extremely satisfied, very satisfied, somewhat satisfied, somewhat dissatisfied, very dissatisfied, or extremely dissatisfied. How would you attempt to summarize all of those scores? You could develop a table (see Table 9.1) that shows the number and percentage of people that endorsed each response. This is one way to describe a **frequency distribution**, which shows how often different scores or values occur for a variable. In viewing the table, you could quickly determine that the vast majority of people appear to be at least somewhat satisfied in their marriage, with about 45% reporting being extremely satisfied.

You could also show the same information using a bar graph (see Figure 9.1) with each bar representing the number or percentage of individuals who endorsed each category. A histogram is another term for a bar graph depicting a frequency distribution. If there are a large number of response categories, then responses can be combined. For example, if you measured marital satisfaction using an instrument like the Dyadic Adjustment Scale (with scores that can range from 0 to 151), then you might graph the scores in 5-point intervals (e.g., 101–105, 106–110).

When researchers examine frequency distributions, they are interested in four properties: (1) measures of central tendency, (2) the variability in scores, (3) the shape of the distribution, and (4) whether there are outliers. Researchers use descriptive statistics to describe the first two properties. Descriptive statistics are helpful because they turn large amounts of data into a manageable form. Using descriptive statistics,

TABLE 9.1. Frequency Table for Marital Satisfaction

Response category	Number	Percentage
Extremely satisfied	180	45.0
Very satisfied	100	25.0
Somewhat satisfied	48	12.0
Somewhat dissatisfied	32	8.0
Very dissatisfied	28	7.0
Extremely dissatisfied	12	3.0

we can take hundreds or even thousands of data points and summarize them in a manner that we can easily grasp. Each of these properties is discussed in more detail below.

Measures of Central Tendency

Researchers often report a **measure of central tendency,** which attempts to capture the value upon which most of the scores are centered. The **mean** or average is the most common way of doing this. The mean is calculated by finding the sum of all the scores, then dividing the sum by the number of scores (see Table 9.2). Means are typically used with ratio

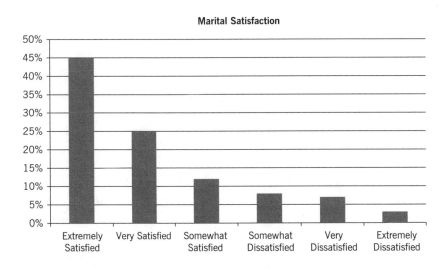

FIGURE 9.1. Histogram, or bar graph, for marital satisfaction.

or interval data, occasionally with ordinal data, but never with nominal data.

The **median** is another measure of central tendency, and represents the middle value if the scores are arranged from lowest to highest (see Table 9.2). If there is an even number of data points, then the median is the mean of the two middle scores. Half of the scores are above the median, and half are below. Like the mean, the median is used with ratio, interval, or ordinal data (but never with nominal data). The median is a better measure of central tendency if there are extreme scores (outliers). This is because extreme scores are less likely to impact the median compared to the mean. In the example depicted in Table 9.2, the mean (2.5) is higher than the median (2.0) because the one student who had a high number of undergraduate research classes is influencing the mean score. Similarly, the news typically reports the median selling price of homes rather than the mean because the mean can be unduly affected by the sale of a small number of very expensive mansions or estates.

The **mode** is a third measure of central tendency, and is the most frequently occurring score (see Table 9.2). If two or more scores tie for being the most frequently occurring score, then each of them is reported as the mode. The mode is the only one appropriate for nominal data, but can be used with ratio, interval, or ordinal data.

Measures of Variability in Scores

There are three ways to measure the variability in scores for a frequency distribution. The simplest is the **range**, which represents the difference between the highest and lowest values (see Table 9.2). However, the range may give a distorted picture if there are extreme scores (outliers). The standard deviation and variance are generally better measures of variability because they are based on all the data points rather than just the highest and lowest scores. Conceptually, the **variance** is similar to finding the average distance of scores from the mean. However, the distance between each score and the mean is squared before finding the average (see Table 9.2). Otherwise, the sum of the scores will be zero because they cancel each other out.[1] The **standard deviation** is simply the square root of the variance (see Table 9.2). The standard deviation

---

[1] The sum of the squared distances is divided by the number of scores when using population values, but it is divided by the number of scores minus one (the degrees of freedom) when using values from a sample of the population.

TABLE 9.2. Illustration for Measures of Central Tendency and Variability

Number of undergraduate research classes 10 students had prior to graduate school:

Adele—2   Carlos—1   Gabby—2   Mary—0   Rhianna—7

Miguel—3   Whitney—1   Tonya—2   Ali—3   Robin—4

Mean = sum of the scores/number of scores:

(2 + 1 + 2 + 0 + 7 + 3 + 1 + 2 + 3 + 4)/10 = 25/10 = 2.5

Median = middle score (average of two middle scores if an even number):

0, 1, 1, 2, 2, 2, 3, 3, 4, 7; Middle score = (2 + 2)/2 = 2

Mode = most frequently occurring score = 2

Range = difference between largest and smallest scores: (7 – 0) = 7

Variance = sum of squares/number of population scores (or $n - 1$ for sample scores):

$(0 - 2.5)^2 = (-2.5)^2 = 6.25$ $(2 - 2.5)^2 = (-0.5)^2 = 0.25$

$(1 - 2.5)^2 = (-1.5)^2 = 2.25$ $(3 - 2.5)^2 = (0.5)^2 = 0.25$

$(1 - 2.5)^2 = (-1.5)^2 = 2.25$ $(3 - 2.5)^2 = (0.5)^2 = 0.25$

$(2 - 2.5)^2 = (-0.5)^2 = 0.25$ $(4 - 2.5)^2 = (1.5)^2 = 2.25$

$(2 - 2.5)^2 = (-0.5)^2 = 0.25$ $(7 - 2.5)^2 = (4.5)^2 = 20.25$

6.25 + 2.25 + 2.25 + 0.25 + 0.25 + 0.25 + 0.25 + 0.25 + 2.25 + 2.25 + 20.25 = 34.5

Sum of squares (34.5) / 10 (number of score for population) = 3.45

Standard deviation = square root of variance = $\sqrt{3.45}$ = 1.86

is typically reported rather than the variance because it is in the same units as the mean.

Shapes of Frequency Distributions

Researchers are often interested in the shape of a frequency distribution. If you constructed a histogram of many phenomena (e.g., IQ scores, height), you will find it often has a bell-shaped curve like the one in Figure 9.2. Researchers refer to this bell-shaped curve as a **normal distribution**.

Normal distributions are important for two reasons. First, if the distribution is normal, then we can convert an individual's absolute score

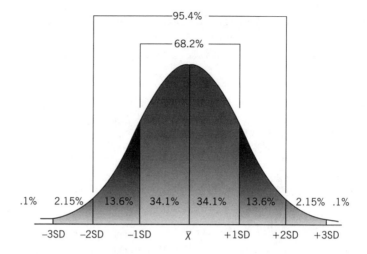

FIGURE 9.2. Normal distribution. $\overline{X}$ = mean, SD = standard deviation. The percentages represent the area under the curve.

into a percentile score. For example, scores on the Graduate Record Exam (GRE) can be converted into a percentile score so you can see how your score compares to others. Different points on the normal distribution correspond with various percentiles, with the mean or average being the 50th percentile (refer to Figure 9.2). Scores one standard deviation above and below the mean correspond to the 84th and 16th percentile, respectively. Thus, a percentile score can be derived based on how many standard deviations the score is above or below the mean. Most scores (68%) will fall within one standard deviation of the mean, while approximately 95% of the scores will fall within two standard deviations of the mean.

  Second, many statistical analyses assume the variables have a normal distribution. If they don't, then the results may not be valid. Not all distributions will be normally distributed. Some may have more scores on the left side (see Figure 9.1), while others may have more on the right. These distributions are described as being **skewed.** If a variable has a skewed distribution, then a mathematical transformation of the scores can be used to make it more normal so it can be used in an analysis.[2]

---

[2] The type of mathematical transformation used depends on the shape of the distribution. For example, a frequency distribution with scores skewed on the left side might be transformed into a normal curve by using the square root of each score. Although mathematical transformations can fix a problem with skewness, they make interpretation of the results more complicated.

Outliers

When researchers examine frequency distributions, they also look for extreme scores called **outliers**. In Figure 9.3, the value to the far right is an outlier. Some outliers result from errors in the data, which need to be corrected. However, in other instances, it may reflect a unique situation or distinct phenomenon. It is even possible that finding an outlier may be an important discovery by identifying an exception to the rule.

APPLICATION

Evaluating Studies

Descriptive statistics are commonly used to summarize demographic or other key variables in a study. You should examine if the researcher used appropriate descriptive statistics for each variable. For example, the researcher should ideally report the median or mode if the variable is skewed or has outliers. The statistic should also be appropriate given the level of measurement for that variable. Also, if means are reported, did the researcher follow the convention of including standard deviations as well?

Many statistical analyses assume the variables have normal distributions. Does the researcher give any indication that the variables were

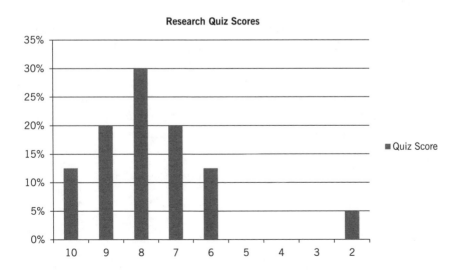

FIGURE 9.3. Example of an outlier.

examined to ensure these conditions were met? Many times this is not included in the report even if the researcher was attentive to this issue. However, if the researcher addresses this issue, then you have greater confidence that the analyses were done in an appropriate manner.

The Normal Distribution in Real Life

The fact that many things in life follow the normal or bell-shaped curve can help remind us what is "normal." Remembering that people's ability may follow a bell-shaped curve can help us be more accepting or patient with others, particularly if we have unrealistically high expectations.[3] For example, we have all encountered drivers who put others at risk through their poor driving. It is easy to fall into a line of thinking that says they "should" be more careful. However, the normal distribution reminds us that we need to expect and accept that a certain percentage of drivers will be poor. Rather than be angry, we should be prepared.

Our own performance may follow a normal distribution, which is a good reminder for those with perfectionistic qualities. Even if we typically perform at a high level, the normal distribution predicts that a certain percentage of time our performance will be on the low end of the distribution. The bell-shaped curve reminds us that we are not always perfect. To err is human or "normal."

Outliers

As therapists, we should also be on the outlook for outliers. Our clients can fall into repetitive patterns that create problems in their lives. However, if one looks carefully, individuals occasionally step outside their normal patterns, resulting in alternative outcomes. Solution-focused therapists call these exceptions. Exceptions are essentially outliers because they fall outside the more common experience of the problem. Searching for these exceptions or outliers can open the door to change.

---

[3] As one supervisor joked, half the people are below average in intelligence.

CHAPTER 10

Inferential Bivariate Statistics

Imagine that your friend wants to demonstrate to you that she has extrasensory powers (ESP). To prove she has ESP, she states that she will accurately predict the color of cards randomly drawn from a shuffled deck. She first predicts that you will turn over a red card, which proves to be correct. Does this prove she has ESP? Probably not given that she had a 50% chance of correctly guessing the card's color. However, your friend goes on to correctly foretell the color of the second and third card. Is she simply lucky three times in a row, or does she really possess ESP? If your friend continues to successfully predict each card's color, at some point you will conclude your friend must have ESP because the odds of correctly guessing the color of so many cards in a row is improbably low and could not simply be due to chance or luck.

Our ESP example parallels how researchers decide if the results they find in samples drawn from a population are a real reflection of what is happening in the population, or are simply an artifact of chance factors that occur during sampling. Chance factors during sampling (sampling error) can create samples that are nonrepresentative of the population. Using inferential statistics, we can calculate the probability that the result we obtained in our sample (e.g., correlations, difference in scores) is due to chance factors or sampling error. This probability is called a p-value, which researchers use to decide if they believe the result is real or an artifact of sampling error.

In our ESP example, at what point do you decide your friend has ESP and her ability to predict is not simply due to chance (e.g., being lucky)? The answer can depend upon each individual. Some might be convinced after she successfully predicts four cards in a row because there is only a 6.25% probability that she could correctly guess this many by chance alone. Others might want to see her get at least seven cards in a row correct because there is less than a 1% chance she could be this lucky simply by guessing.

In a similar manner, researchers must decide how conservative they will be before concluding the sample result is a real reflection of what exists in the population and is not due to chance factors. Most researchers will not assume the sample result is real unless the probability that it could be due to chance is 5% (.05) or less. Others are more conservative, and may insist that the probability not be more than 1% (or .01). If the p-value is less than the chosen level of significance (e.g., .05 or .01), then the result is said to be statistically significant. In other words, the sample results are presumed to hold true for the population, and are not simply an artifact of sampling error.

As you will read in this chapter, statistical significance is not the same as clinical significance. A small, but statistically significant difference may not be of large enough magnitude to be of practical or clinical significance. We must consider both statistical and clinical significance when evaluating results from studies.

THE BASICS OF INFERENTIAL STATISTICS

Sampling Error and Inferential Statistics

In Chapter 4 we discussed that it is often impractical to collect information from an entire population. To address this problem, researchers draw a sample using probability sampling that they hope is representative of the population. However, chance or random factors may result in the sample not being 100% representative, which researchers refer to as **sampling error**. If you want a firsthand experience with sampling error, take a coin and flip it 10 times, and then record the number of heads that you obtain. Repeat this process nine more times to create 10 samples. If you construct a histogram of your results, you may get a distribution that resembles the one in Figure 10.1. If a sample is representative of the population of coin flips, then you should get five heads because 50% of the coin flips should result in heads. However, you will notice that this is not always the case. In our example, only four of the samples had the expected five heads. The other six samples had either more or less than

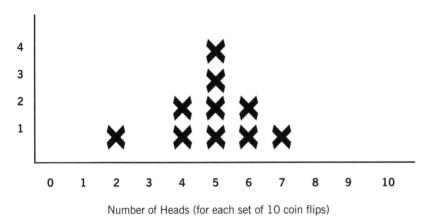

FIGURE 10.1. Histogram for coin-flip example.

five heads. One sample had only two heads. In some cases, you may even get a sample with all heads or no heads at all. This is all a result of sampling error.

Small samples are more likely to suffer from sampling error because chance factors are less likely to cancel out. The likelihood of getting all heads with three coin flips is much greater than getting all heads with 10 coin flips. You can observe this effect with the coin samples you collected. If you count the number of heads across all 100 of your coin flips, you will notice that the number is probably close to 50, or 50%. For example, the total number of heads in Figure 10.1 is 49 (out of 100 coin flips), which is very close to the 50% we would expect. Thus, a sample of 100 is more likely to give an accurate picture than a sample of 10. This is why, as you will see later on, it is easier to get statistically significant results with larger samples because sampling error is smaller.

Inferential statistics help us take into account sampling error when drawing conclusions about a population based on findings from our sample. We might use inferential statistics to help us predict a value in the population based on our sample (e.g., the percentage of individuals who vote for each candidate). Or, inferential statistics can help us evaluate the probability that the results we observe in a sample are simply an artifact of sampling error. If this probability is low, then we will conclude the relationship is likely a real reflection of what exists in the population. We will now turn our attention to describing how to use inferential statistics in both of these cases.

Estimating Population Values

Polls are familiar to nearly everyone. During election season, the news will often report poll results that predict the winner of upcoming elections. Polls may also be used to estimate what percentage of the population holds a particular view or opinion.

The accuracy of a poll depends upon how representative the sample is of the larger population. A poll conducted solely among college students may not be representative of the general population. It also depends on how large the sample is. As we described above, a small sample is more likely to suffer from sampling error.

If we attempt to obtain a representative sample of the population through probability sampling, we can use the values from the sample to predict the population values. Due to sampling error, the sample values may not precisely reflect the population values. However, researchers can predict with some confidence that the population value will fall within a certain range based on their knowledge of the sample such as its size and the variation of scores in the sample (e.g., standard deviation). With this information, researchers can predict with 95% confidence that the actual population value falls within a certain range known as the **confidence interval**. The confidence interval is also called the **margin of error**. Thus, a poll may indicate that 52% of individuals will cast their vote for a particular candidate, and that the poll has a margin of error of ±3 points. In other words, the pollster can state with 95% confidence that the actual percentage in the population will be between 49% and 55%. Larger samples will result in smaller confidence intervals or margins of error because sampling error will be less.

Bivariate Statistics and Statistical Significance

When we observe a relationship between two variables in a sample, there are two possible explanations. The first explanation is that the observed relationship does not reflect a real relationship in the population, but is simply an artifact of sampling error. Researchers call this the **null hypothesis**. The alternative explanation, which researchers have creatively called the **alternative hypothesis**, is that the observed relationship in the sample reflects a relationship that really exists in the population.

Inferential statistics help us evaluate which hypothesis may be true. Each of the statistical tests we will describe below calculates a statistic (e.g., t-test, chi-square) and a corresponding p-value. The **p-value** represents the probability that the observed relationship in the sample could be due to sampling error. Based on the p-value, we can then decide whether we think the null hypothesis or the alternative hypothesis is true. If we decide the alternative hypothesis is true, then we have concluded that the result is **statistically significant**.

How low the p-value must be before we reject the null hypothesis and assume the alternative hypothesis is true is a matter of judgment. The required p-value to reject the null hypothesis and assume the alternative hypothesis is true is called the **level of significance**, or **alpha**. The most common convention is to use .05 as the level of significance. In other words, the p-value must be .05 or less before we reject the null hypothesis and assume the alternative hypothesis is true. Other researchers may be more conservative and require that the p-value be .01 or less to achieve statistical significance.[1] In some cases, the researcher may relax the level of significance to .10 if the study has a small sample and is exploratory in nature. Researchers often report the actual p-value so readers can decide for themselves whether the findings are statistically significant based on their own preferred level of significance.

Because statistical significance is based on a probability statement, there are four possible outcomes (see Figure 10.2). The researcher could either correctly conclude the null hypothesis is true when it is indeed true, or reject the null hypothesis when the alternative hypothesis is true. However, there is the potential to make two wrong decisions. The first potential error is to reject the null hypothesis and assume the observed relationship in the sample is real, but in actuality the relationship is an artifact of sampling error. Researchers call this a **Type I error**. To minimize Type I error, researchers typically set the level of significance low (.05 or .01). However, this increases the likelihood of making a **Type II error**, which is to assume that the sample result is simply an artifact of sampling error, but in reality it exists in the population.

An everyday example can illustrate Type I and Type II errors and the trade-off between the two. If the weather forecast states there is a 30% chance of rain, you must decide if it will rain and whether to take your umbrella or not. If you take your umbrella assuming that it will rain, then you made the correct decision if it later rains. However, if you assume it will rain and it does not, then you made a Type I error, which results in you needlessly carrying your umbrella around all day. You will

---

[1]You can also think of the p-value as a percentage. Thus, a .05 level of significance would be equivalent to a 5% probability that the null hypothesis is true. Likewise, a .01 level of significance would be equivalent to a 1% probability that the null hypothesis is true.

	Population	
	Null Is True	Null Is False
Decision Based on Sample		
Reject Null (Null Is False)	Type I Error	Correct Decision
Accept Null as True	Correct Decision	Type II Error

FIGURE 10.2. Four possible outcomes for rejecting or accepting the null hypothesis.

leave the umbrella at home if you assume that it will not rain, which will be the correct judgment if it never rains. However, if you assume that it will not rain and it later does, then you made a Type II error, with the unfortunate result of you being caught in the rain without an umbrella.

There is a trade-off between the two potential errors. If you hate to get caught in the rain without an umbrella, you are likely to take your umbrella even if there is a small chance of rain (e.g., 10%). Although this minimizes your risk of getting unexpectedly wet, it also increases the likelihood that you will be carrying an umbrella around on days that it never rains. Conversely, if you dislike toting umbrellas around, then you will be more willing to leave the umbrella at home to spare yourself the aggravation of carrying and perhaps losing your umbrella. However, you will also be more likely to get caught in the rain without an umbrella.

As our umbrella example illustrates, individuals may dislike making one error more than the other. Researchers try to avoid concluding something is real when it is not (Type I error) by setting the level of significance at .05 or .01. However, being conservative in this regard increases the likelihood of assuming a result is due to sampling error, when in fact it is real (Type II error). We will revisit this issue in the application section when we explore how the two types of errors can impact decision making.

Bivariate Statistics

A number of bivariate statistical tests are used to help us evaluate the likelihood that a relationship between two variables is real or due to sampling error. Determining which test to use depends upon the nature of the relationship and the level of measurement (see Chapter 2) for each variable. The most common bivariate analyses you will read about are summarized in Table 10.1. Each of these analyses is described in more detail below.

The **chi-square** (χ^2) test is used to determine if there is a relationship between two categorical variables. For example, a chi-square analysis would be used to determine if there is a relationship between receiving marriage preparation (yes/no) and the couple's marital status (married/divorced) after 10 years. The chi-square is the only test that can be used to determine if there is a relationship between two nominal variables. It can also be used for ordinal variables, particularly if there are a limited number of categories. Chi-square analyses only evaluate whether a relationship exists or not, and not the strength of the relationship. Separate correlational analyses (e.g., lambda, Cramér's V) are used to measure the strength of the relationship if the chi-square is found to be significant.

Pearson's r correlation is used to evaluate if a relationship exists between two continuous variables (interval or ratio level of measurement) and the strength of the relationship. It also tells you the direction of the relationship based on whether the correlation coefficient is positive or negative. Positive correlations indicate that increasing values of one variable (x) are associated with increasing values of another variable (y). The amount of time studying for an exam should be positively related to the exam score. A negative correlation means that increasing values of x are associated with decreasing values of y. One would anticipate a

TABLE 10.1. Common Bivariate Statistical Analyses

Name	Purpose of the analysis
Chi-square	Does a significant relationship exist between two categorical variables?
Pearson's r correlation	Does a significant relationship exist between two continuous variables? The Pearson's r also indicates the strength and the direction of the relationship.
t-test	Is the mean score for a dependent variable (continuous) significantly different between *two* groups (categorical variable)?
ANOVA	Is the mean score for a dependent variable (continuous) significantly different across *two or more* groups (categorical variable)?

negative correlation between the amount of conflict in the relationship and relationship satisfaction.

Pearson's r correlations can range between zero and one, and can be either positive or negative. A correlation of zero means there is no relationship between the two variables. A correlation of one (positive or negative) means there is a perfect one-to-one association between the two variables. In the next chapter we will discuss how squaring the Pearson r coefficient gives you a measure of how well values of x predict values of y.

Pearson's r can be influenced by a number of factors. Pearson's r will not accurately measure the strength of association if the variables are not linearly related, such as a curvilinear relationship (see Figure 10.3a). Outliers can also inflate or deflate the strength of correlations. For example, in Figure 10.3b, three outliers make what would be an otherwise weak correlation appear to be stronger than it really is. Conversely, Figure 10.3c shows how outliers can make a modest correlation appear weaker

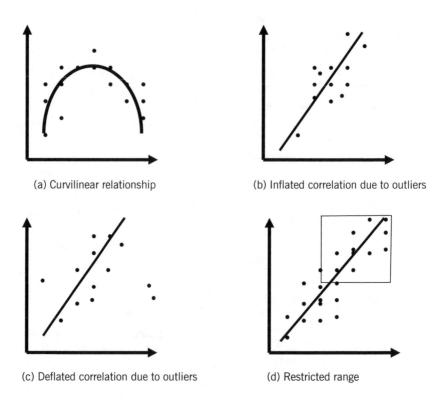

(a) Curvilinear relationship

(b) Inflated correlation due to outliers

(c) Deflated correlation due to outliers

(d) Restricted range

FIGURE 10.3. Factors that impact correlations.

than it really is. That is why it is important for researchers to inspect the frequency distributions for outliers (see Chapter 9). Finally, correlations may not be accurate if the phenomenon is measured over a restricted range. If you look at Figure 10.3d, you will notice that the correlation within the box (the restricted range) does not appear as strong when compared to the correlation that uses all the data points.

Although Pearson's r is the most commonly reported correlation, it is just one of the many types of correlations (see Table 10.2). The appropriate correlation depends upon the level of measurement of the variables.

The **t-test** is another commonly used inferential statistic, and is used to evaluate whether the mean scores between two groups are different. A t-test might be used to evaluate if the mean Beck Depression Inventory score between a cognitive-behavioral treatment (CBT) group and a no-treatment control group are different.

An **ANOVA (analysis of variance)** can also be used to measure if the mean scores are different between groups. Unlike the t-test, which is restricted to comparing two groups, ANOVAs can compare two or more groups. Therefore, we could use an ANOVA to see if the Beck depression scores are different between groups that received CBT, medication, and a no-treatment control. If a statistically significant result is found, the researcher will need to do a subsequent **post-hoc analysis** to determine which groups are different from one another. That is because an ANOVA only indicates if a significant difference exists between any of the groups, but not specifically which ones. In order to determine which groups are different from one another, a post-hoc analysis such as the Scheffé, Newman–Keuls, or Duncan multiple range would need to be

TABLE 10.2. Different Types of Correlations and Their Level of Measurement

	Level of measurement	
Type of correlation	Variable x	Variable y
Lambda Cramér's V Phi	Nominal	Nominal
Spearman's rho Kendall's tau Gamma	Ordinal	Ordinal
Pearson's r	Interval/ratio	Interval/ratio

run. For example, it could be the CBT and medication groups are not significantly different from each other, but the no-treatment control group is different from both.

The logic of interpreting bivariate statistics is similar across analyses (see Table 10.3). You can determine which test was conducted by looking at the reported statistic. For example, a t-value will be reported for a t-test and an F-value for an ANOVA. The number in parentheses is the degrees of freedom (df).[2] After the equal sign, the calculated value for the statistic will be reported. However, the reader will generally be more interested in the p-value that is provided next, which is used to determine if the result is statistically significant. If the p-value is equal to or less than our level of significance, then we reject the null hypothesis and assume the alternative hypothesis is true.

Statistical versus Clinical Significance

It is important to distinguish between statistical and clinical significance. **Clinical significance** relates to whether the result is of practical significance. Results that are statistically significant are not automatically clinically significant. Imagine that a study for treating anorexia nervosa shows a statistically significant difference between a treatment and no-treatment group in terms of weight gain. However, if the average weight gain for the treatment group is only three pounds higher than the control group, is this big enough to be of clinical significance? In other words, is it a large enough difference to improve the health of severely underweight individuals? In the application section, we will discuss how to evaluate if results are clinically significant.

APPLICATION

Evaluating Inferential Statistics

How can you know if the inferential statistics have been done correctly? As we discussed in the previous chapter, many statistical analyses make certain assumptions about the variables used in the analysis. These can include the absence of outliers and having a normal distribution. Unfortunately, researchers rarely make explicit that they confirmed these

---

[2] A detailed description of degrees of freedom is outside the scope of this book. However, for many analyses, it is related to the number of observations. For example, the Pearson's r correlation has $N - 2$ degrees of freedom, where N is the number of paired comparisons.

TABLE 10.3. Interpreting Statistical Results

Type of test	Statistic	Degrees of freedom	Calculated value	p-value
Chi-square	χ^2	(1)	= 3.84;	$p = .05$
Pearson's r correlation	r	(25)	= -.49;	$p = .01$
t-test	t	(18)	= 1.73;	$p = .10$
ANOVA	F	(2, 40)	= 5.18;	$p = .01$

assumptions were met before running their analyses. However, your confidence in a researcher's competence is enhanced if he or she acknowledges that these assumptions were examined.

It is important to note that using inferential statistics assumes the sample was drawn from the population using probability sampling (see Chapter 4). However, inferential statistics are frequently used on data sets collected by convenience sampling. Therefore, the use of inferential statistics should not make us overlook that the type of sampling used also impacts our ability to generalize from a sample to a population. This may be less of a concern for exploratory work that is simply attempting to explore what relationships may exist between different variables. However, convenience sampling undermines one's ability to accurately estimate population values even when using inferential statistics.

Statistical versus Clinical Significance

Ideally, researchers will address the issue of clinical significance in reporting their results, but this is often not the case. For studies that include comparison between groups (e.g., experimental studies, meta-analyses), the effect size can be used to judge the clinical significance of the findings. As stated in Chapter 7 when discussing meta-analysis, an effect size around 0.20 is weak, medium if around 0.50, and strong if 0.80 and above (Cohen, 1988).

If Pearson's r correlations are reported, then you can examine the strength of the correlation as a measure of clinical significance. For example, a study with a large sample size may report that a correlation of .11 is statistically significant. However, the size of this correlation is weak. As a general guideline, Cohen (1988) has suggested that correlations (r statistic) are small at .10, medium at .30, and large if .50 and above.

Clinical significance can be expressed in other ways, such as odds ratios or risk ratios. Odds ratios (OR) and risk ratios (also referred to as relative risk) compare the likelihood of an event happening in one group compared to the likelihood of it happening in another group. For example, an odds ratio can tell us if individuals are more likely to divorce based on whether they cohabitated or not. Odds ratios and risk ratios above 1 means the event is more likely to occur in the first group compared to the second group. Odds ratios and risk ratios less than 1 indicate the event is more likely to occur in the second group. According to Rutledge and Loh (2004), odds ratios and risk ratios are a better indicator of clinical significance than correlations when both the predictor and outcome variables are dichotomous, and the incidence of the outcome event (e.g., contracting a disease, developing a side effect) is small. That is because even a significant change in the occurrence of an infrequent event (e.g., doubling of 1% to 2%) will still result in a small correlation because the incidence of the event is still small.

Another approach to establishing clinical significance is to report the percentage of individuals that deteriorated, did not change, improved, and fully recovered. The fully recovered group would represent those who scored in the functional range on an established measure. For example, a study that evaluated a treatment for marital distress would report the percentage of couples whose scores on the Dyadic Adjustment Scale were above the cutoff for nondistressed couples.

Type I and Type II Error in Decision Making

Like researchers who must decide whether to accept or reject the null hypothesis based on a probability (the p-value), there are situations in life that require we make a judgment based on a probability that it might be true. For example, a jury must decide whether a person accused of a crime is guilty or not. Before finding the defendant guilty, they must assess if the evidence against the individual is greater than reasonable doubt. Similar to Figure 10.2, there are four possible outcomes based on the jury's decision. The jury may correctly determine if the individual is guilty or innocent. They could also make two types of errors—deciding the defendant is guilty when he or she is innocent, or deciding the defendant is innocent when he or she is guilty.

Our values can impact which type of error we most want to avoid. For example, our legal system is based on the value that it is worse to convict an innocent person than to let a guilty individual go. As a result, our legal system has established procedures (e.g., reasonable doubt, complete consensus for a jury) to minimize this type of error.

When we (or our clients) are making difficult decisions based on probabilities, it may be helpful to examine our values and how they might inform our decision making. What are the consequences of making one type of error, and how do they compare with the consequences of making the other type of error? Stefan found himself facing this dilemma. He suspected that Brooke had an affair based on some weak, circumstantial evidence. However, he lacked conclusive evidence and Brooke denied having an affair. The couple became trapped in a vicious cycle around the issue. When Stefan would express his suspicions, Brooke would become hurt and distance herself from him. However, her distancing only reinforced Stefan's fears that she had been unfaithful. The couple seemed at an impasse, particularly because there was no way for Stefan to know for sure whether Brooke indeed had an affair.

In an attempt to break the vicious cycle, the therapist helped Stefan map out the four possible outcomes and the possible consequences associated with each outcome. For example, if Brooke had been faithful and he believed her, then he would be making a good decision. They also explored the possible mistakes that could arise: (1) believing Brooke's claim that she was faithful, when in reality she did have an affair, and (2) assuming Brooke had an affair when she had actually remained faithful. He was asked to think about what making each mistake would mean to him. For example, Stefan stated he would feel foolish if he believed Brooke and later learned that she actually had an affair. The opposite mistake would be to wrongly assume Brooke had an affair, and let his distrust and anger destroy the relationship. Stefan was next encouraged to think about which mistake would have the most serious consequences for him. After reflection, Stefan decided he would rather give Brooke the benefit of the doubt because the relationship was more important to him than later feeling foolish if he discovered she had had an affair. Recognizing this helped Stefan become unstuck.

CHAPTER 11

A Beginner's Guide
to Multivariate Statistics

You have just been offered a job at company XYZ. Before accepting the offer, you weigh a number of factors to determine if you will be happy working for them. For example, you consider things such as the salary, amount of vacation time, the opportunity for promotion, and how much you like the person who will be your boss. From a research perspective, you are doing a multivariate analysis by looking at how multiple factors (e.g., salary, vacation time) relate to an outcome variable (job satisfaction).

Life is complicated. That is why we need **multivariate statistics**. Multivariate statistics allow us to consider if two or more factors are related to a particular outcome. The analysis that is done depends upon the type of variables we use to predict the outcome, as well as the outcome variable. For example, if you simply want to predict if you will be happy with the job, which is dichotomous (yes/no), then you will use one method. If you want to predict an outcome that can range in value, such as level of job satisfaction, then this will require using a different multivariate analysis. The next section will describe various multivariate analyses commonly used in psychotherapy research.

THE FUNDAMENTALS
OF MULTIVARIATE STATISTICS

Multiple Regression

If two variables correlate with one another, then you can use one to predict the other. For example, if SAT scores correlate with college GPAs, then we can predict an individual's college GPA if we know his or her SAT score. A variable used to predict another variable is called an **independent variable**, while the outcome variable is called the **dependent variable**. In this example, the independent variable is SAT scores and the dependent variable is college GPA.

The stronger the correlation is between two variables, the better the independent variable will be at predicting scores for the dependent variable. Squaring the Pearson's r correlation is an indication of how well the independent variable predicts the dependent variable. Hypothetically, if SAT scores have a .50 correlation with college GPAs, then SAT scores will explain or account for 25% of the variation in college GPAs (.50 × .50 = .25 or 25%). This means 75% of the remaining variance is explained by other variables. Hence, including other variables may improve our ability to predict a student's college GPA. This is precisely why we need multiple regression.

Multiple regression allows us to use more than one independent variable to predict a dependent variable. For example, rather than rely just on SAT scores to predict college GPAs, we might also include high school GPAs. If the high school GPA correlates with the college GPA, then adding this variable to our equation may give us a more accurate prediction of a student's college GPA. The two variables will ideally have a stronger correlation collectively than either one by itself. The correlation between the independent variables and the dependent variable is called **multiple R**, and it can range from 0 (no correlation) to 1 (a perfect correlation).

If you square multiple R like we did with the Pearson's r correlation, then we will know how well the independent variables collectively predict the dependent variable. If multiple R is .70 in our hypothetical example, then R^2 tells us that SAT scores and high school GPAs predict 49% of the variance (.70 × .70 = .49, or 49%) in college GPAs. This means about half (51%) of the variance is still unaccounted for, which suggests that other variables may impact college GPAs. In multiple regression, we can add additional variables to see if we can strengthen our ability to predict something.

In multiple regression, the independent variables are primarily continuous variables (interval or ratio levels of measurement), although dichotomous variables can also be used (e.g., yes/no). The dependent variable is continuous (interval or ratio) in multiple regression. Other analyses such as discriminant function analysis or logistic regression (discussed below) are used if the dependent variable is categorical rather than continuous.

A researcher has three options on how to enter independent variables into a multiple regression analysis. They are **standard** (or simultaneous), **hierarchical** (or sequential), or **stepwise**. An example of each option is illustrated below.

Standard multiple regression, sometimes called simultaneous multiple regression, puts all of the independent variables into the analysis at one time. You can assume the researcher used the standard method unless otherwise specified. Table 11.1 shows what the results from a standard multiple regression might look like using a hypothetical example. In our example, the researcher is attempting to predict therapist confidence (the dependent variable) based on five independent variables: (1) the number of client contact hours, (2) the number of positive critical incidences the therapist has experienced with clients, (3) the number of supervision hours received, (4) scores from an index that measures the therapist's level of perfectionism, and (5) the therapist's age.

When reviewing the results of a standard multiple regression, you will want to examine the values for multiple R and R^2. These will help you assess how good the independent variables are collectively in predicting the dependent variable. In our example, multiple R is .61, with a corresponding R^2 of .37. This means that our five independent variables collectively can predict 37% of the variance. The results may also include an adjusted R^2 value, which compensates for chance factors that may inflate R^2 based on sample size and the number of independent variables.

It can also be important to know which variables are the most powerful predictors. To determine this, you will typically want to look at the beta coefficients (ß) for each independent variable. Beta coefficients are like correlations, with higher absolute values representing a stron-

TABLE 11.1. Standard Multiple Regression Example: Predicting Therapist Confidence

Variable	B	SE B	Beta (ß)
Client contact hours	.009	.003	.21**
Positive critical incidences	.520	.22	.25**
Supervision hours	.016	.007	.11*
Perfectionism Index	−.360	.14	−.09*
Age	−.003	.001	−.02
(Constant)	.159		

Multiple R = .61; R^2 = .37; adjusted R^2 = .35.
**$p \leq .01$; *$p \leq .05$.

ger relationship. The variables with the highest beta coefficients will be the strongest predictors. Thus, in our example, the number of positive critical incidences in therapy is the strongest predictor of therapist confidence ($\beta = .25$), followed by client contact hours ($\beta = .21$), supervision hours ($\beta = .11$) and perfectionism ($\beta = -.09$). Age, the fifth variable, does not appear to be a predictor of therapist confidence because it was not statistically significant in the analysis. Sometimes a squared semi-partial correlation (sr^2) will be reported for each variable, which can be used instead of beta coefficients to determine the relative importance of an independent variable.[1]

Beta coefficients also have positive or negative values indicating the direction of the relationship. Thus, higher values on the first three variables (client contact hours, number of positive incidences, supervision hours) are all associated with higher therapist confidence. In contrast, higher scores for perfectionism are associated with lower therapist confidence.

Researchers will also report a regression coefficient (B or b) for each independent variable, along with its corresponding standard error term (SE B). The regression coefficients and the constant can be used in a multiple regression equation to predict the dependent variable based on new values for the independent variables. Typically, predicting scores for the dependent variable using the regression equation is not as critical in the psychotherapy field as understanding which variables are the most important predictors. However, in some fields like economics, being able to predict these values is important.

If the variables are entered using the hierarchical (or sequential) method, then they are entered in sets according to the researcher's preferences. The order is usually determined by theory. For example, Williams (1995) tested a stress–vulnerability model for predicting marital satisfaction using hierarchical multiple regression. Factors that were measured during the couple's engagement and hypothesized to reflect a preexisting vulnerability were entered in the first set. The stress subsequently experienced in the marriage was added in the second set to see if it enhanced the ability to predict marital satisfaction. By comparing the R^2 values between each set, you can determine how much additional explanatory power the new set of variables adds. In the above example,

---

[1]Squared semi-partial correlations (sr^2) may actually give a more accurate picture of the relative importance of independent variables because of the way they account for shared variance among variables.

the vulnerability variables yielded an R^2 of .157 for women. Adding stress experienced during the marriage in the second set improved R^2 to .190. The difference (.190 – .157 = .033) indicates that adding stress helped to account for an additional 3.3% of the variance.

Stepwise is a third way to enter variables into a multiple regression analysis. In this approach, independent variables enter one at a time according to their ability to predict the dependent variable. The statistical program selects the most powerful predictor and enters it first. The next most powerful predictor is selected and entered in the second step. This process continues until all of the significant predictor variables have been entered. Table 11.2 shows a hypothetical example of a stepwise multiple regression used to predict performance on a research methods final exam. In this example, time spent studying for the final exam was the best predictor of the final exam score, so it was entered first. The next best predictor of final exam scores was the midterm scores for students, so it was entered in the second step. Two other variables (SAT mathematics scores, math anxiety scores) are added in the subsequent two steps based on their ability to predict final exam scores. In stepwise analyses, some variables may never be added if they do not contribute significantly to the equation's ability to predict the dependent variable. In our example, SAT reading scores and writing scores do not significantly predict the final exam scores for the research class, so they are never added.

In a stepwise regression the multiple R and R^2 will be reported after each step. By comparing the R^2 values between each step, you can determine how much explanatory power was gained by adding each new variable. For example, time spent studying for the final explains 25% ($R^2 = .25$) of the variance by itself. However, adding the midterm score in the second step increases R^2 to .36, which means an additional 11% (.11) of the variance is explained by adding this variable. The R^2 for the last

TABLE 11.2. Stepwise Multiple Regression Example: Predicting Research Final Exam Scores

Step	Variable	Multiple R	R^2	Change in R^2
1	Time spent studying for final	.50	.25	.25
2	Midterm score	.60	.36	.11
3	SAT mathematics score	.66	.44	.08
4	Math anxiety score	.70	.49	.05

Note. Variables that were not entered: SAT reading score, SAT writing score.

step represents the explanatory power for all of the significant variables entered into the equation, which is 49% (or .49) in our example. When evaluating the relative importance of the independent variables, they will be entered in order of most to least powerful by virtue of how the stepwise analysis is conducted.

Discriminant Function Analysis

In the earlier stress–vulnerability example, multiple regression was used to predict marital satisfaction scores, which is a continuous variable. However, a different type of analysis is required if your dependent variable is categorical. **Discriminant function analysis (DFA)** is used if the dependent variable is categorical and all of the independent variables are continuous. (We will discuss logistic regression shortly, which can be used if some of the independent variables are not continuous.) For example, DFA would be used if we wanted to predict whether individuals remained married or divorced after 5 years using the stress–vulnerability model. DFA can help us answer which variables are important in predicting group membership (e.g., married, divorced).

Like multiple regression, DFA generates a correlation between the independent variables and the dependent variable. In DFA, this correlation is called a canonical correlation. Instead of squaring this correlation, the predictive ability of DFA is determined by comparing the group membership predicted by the DFA equation with the actual group membership. If the DFA has good predictive ability, there will be a strong correspondence between the predicted and actual group membership. For example, one study used DFA to evaluate the predictive validity of a premarital inventory called FOCCUS (Williams & Jurich, 1995). Scores from the various topic areas that FOCCUS assesses (e.g., communication, problem solving, financial issues, religion and values) were the independent variables used to predict the couple's marital success 4–5 years after taking the FOCCUS inventory. Couples were categorized as either having a high-quality or poor-quality marriage based on their Dyadic Adjustment Scale (DAS) scores and marital status.[2] Among the couples who later had a high-quality marriage, the DFA correctly predicted 69.2% of these couples would have a high-quality marriage based

---

[2]Couples who were divorced were put into the poor marital quality category along with couples where one or both partners scored in the distressed range on the DAS.

on their FOCCUS scores. Likewise, the DFA correctly classified 76.1% of the couples with low-quality marriages based on their FOCCUS scores. When looking at both high- and low-quality marriages, the DFA equation was able to predict with 73.9% accuracy the future marital quality of couples based on their premarital inventory scores. Therefore, the results support the predictive validity of FOCCUS.

Logistic Regression

Logistic regression is similar to DFA in that it uses multiple independent variables to predict a categorical (nominal) dependent variable. However, logistic regression is different from DFA in that it can use both continuous and categorical variables as independent variables.[3] For example, logistic regression could be used to predict individuals' later marital status (divorced or married) based on a variety of premarital variables such as level of conflict (continuous), level of cohesion (continuous), whether the couple had premarital counseling (categorical), or whether the couple cohabitated before marriage (categorical).

Logistic regression uses logarithms to calculate the odds ratio between the independent variables and the dependent variable.[4] Odds ratios less than 1 indicate that changes in the independent variables are associated with decreased odds or likelihood of the outcome occurring, while odds ratios above 1 are associated with increased odds or likelihood of the outcome occurring. In addition to reporting the odds-ratio for each variable, results from a logistic regression may include the corresponding Wald value and its level of significance so you can determine if the odds ratio is significantly different from 1.0 (which represents no association between the independent and dependent variable). It may also include the 95% confidence level for the odds ratio, which means there is a 95% probability that the actual odds ratio falls inside this range. Like multiple regression, variables can be entered all at once (standard or direct), hierarchically (sequentially), or stepwise.

---

[3] If only categorical (nominal) independent variables are used as predictors, this type of analysis is sometimes called *logit*.

[4] The odds ratio is the odds of an event happening in one group or condition divided by the odds of the event happening in a second group or condition. The odds of the event for each group or condition are calculated by dividing the probability of the event happening (p) by the probability of it not happening ($1 - p$).

Canonical Correlation

In **canonical correlation**, multiple independent variables are used to predict multiple dependent variables. Bowser, Word, Stanton, and Coleman (2003) used canonical correlation to see if there was a relationship between the death of family members and HIV risk taking among intravenous drug users. The results showed that multiple independent variables associated with the loss of a family member (e.g., number of close family member deaths, effectiveness at mourning losses, emotional closeness to family member, funeral attendance) were strongly related to multiple indicators of HIV risk taking (e.g., sexual practices, frequency of drug use, practices when using syringes), the dependent variables. The authors concluded that unresolved grief issues should be assessed and treated when working with intravenous drug users and their families.

Path Analysis and Structural Equation Modeling

Path analysis can be used to study the interrelationship between multiple variables. In path analysis, variables can be both an independent and a dependent variable depending upon their relationship to other variables. The interrelationship between variables is analyzed using a combination of multiple regression analyses. Figure 11.1 is an example of a hypothetical path analysis that looks at the relationship between four variables: (1) understanding research concepts, (2) interest in reading research articles, (3) interest in doing research, and (4) an ability to apply research clinically. The numbers next to the arrows are path coefficients, which are similar to correlations and show the strength and direction of the relationship between the two variables. In this example, understanding research is positively related to both an interest in reading research (.45) and doing research (.25). There is also a positive relationship between having an interest in reading research and one's ability to clinically apply research (.59). However, an interest in doing research did not translate into a significantly stronger ability to apply research clinically (.07), although it may strengthen one's interest in reading research (.53), indirectly contributing to one's ability to apply research clinically.

Researchers interested in looking at the interrelationship between constructs can use an even more sophisticated approach called **structural equation modeling (SEM)**. In path analysis, only one measure

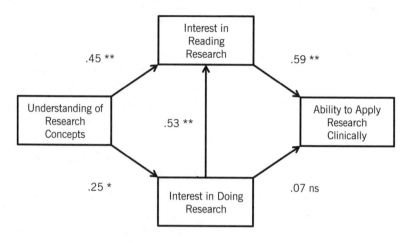

FIGURE 11.1. Hypothetical path analysis example. $^*p < .05$; $^{**}p < .01$.

or scale is used to operationalize each construct. However, SEM uses multiple measures to operationalize each construct. For example, a child's problematic behaviors may be measured using parent reports, teacher reports, and child self-reports. Factor analysis is used to combine the scores from these multiple measures to generate values for each construct. These scores are then analyzed using multiple regression in a manner similar to path analysis to generate an interrelationship between constructs. In SEM, the diagram not only shows the correlation between the constructs, but how strongly each measure relates to the corresponding construct (see Figure 11.2). Researchers will sometimes make reference to special software packages they use to do SEM analyses, such as LISREL, AMOS, or EQS.

ANOVA-Type Analyses

We first introduced you to ANOVA in the previous chapter on bivariate statistics. In this chapter we will discuss how ANOVA and related analyses are used in a multivariate way.

Analysis of Variance

In the last chapter we described ANOVA as a way of seeing if the mean scores for a dependent variable were significantly different between

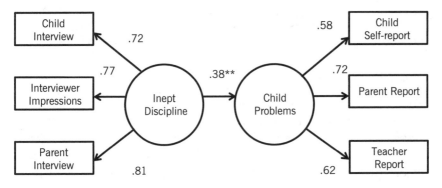

FIGURE 11.2. Simple structural equation modeling diagram. $^{**}p < .01$.

two or more groups. For example, we discussed how ANOVA could be used in an experimental design to see if the average depression scores (the dependent variable) were different based on the type of treatment received (the independent variable), which might have two or more levels (e.g., medication, cognitive-behavioral therapy, or no-treatment control). This is an example of where the ANOVA is a bivariate analysis.

ANOVA can be turned into a multivariate analysis by adding additional independent variables. Perhaps you anticipate the effectiveness of the treatment will depend not only upon the type of treatment received, but also the gender of the individual. Experiments analyzed with ANOVA in this manner are sometimes called **factorial designs**. In our example, the researcher used a 3 × 2 factorial design, where each number represents an independent variable and its corresponding number of levels. Type of treatment has three levels (medication, cognitive therapy, and no-treatment), and gender has two levels (male and female). If we added a third independent variable (presence or absence of suicidal ideation), then we would have a 3 × 2 × 2 factorial design.

A factorial design allows us to not only study if there is a significant difference in scores between each variable (called a *main effect*), but it also allows us to see if the independent variables interact together in having an effect on the dependent variable (called an *interaction effect*). For example, we could see if the average depression score is different based on whether individuals received cognitive-behavioral therapy or medication, a main effect. We could also see if depression scores were different based on gender, a second main effect. Furthermore, we could see if the effectiveness of either cognitive-behavioral therapy or medication depended upon the individual's gender, resulting in an interaction effect.

Analysis of Covariance

Analysis of covariance (ANCOVA) is like ANOVA, except it allows for one of the independent variables to be continuous rather than categorical. For example, ANCOVA could control for the fact that not all subjects have equal pretest scores, with pretest scores being the covariate. In this example, the covariate is like a handicap score in golf where each person's skill level is taken into account when comparing the scores across golfers for a particular game.

Multivariate Analysis of Variance

Multivariate analysis of variance (MANOVA) examines the relationship between a single independent variable that is categorical and multiple dependent variables. MANOVA allows the researcher to test if the mean scores for multiple dependent variables are different for individuals who belong to different groups (independent variable). For example, Jewell and Stark (2003) were interested in knowing if there was a difference in scores for seven family environmental variables (the dependent variables) based on whether or not youth were diagnosed with conduct disorder or major depression (the independent variable). They obtained a statistically significant result for the overall multivariate MANOVA analysis. Follow-up t-tests on each of the dependent variables revealed significant differences on two of the family environmental measures—Enmeshment and Laissez-Faire Family Style (permissive and inconsistent discipline style). Youth who were diagnosed with conduct disorder had significantly higher scores than depressed adolescents on the Laissez-Faire Family Style scale, but significantly lower scores on the Enmeshment scale. Based on these findings, the authors suggest different forms of interventions are necessary for these two groups.

APPLICATION

Evaluating Multivariate Statistics in Research

Evaluating multivariate statistics may be more difficult to assess than other areas we have discussed. However, there are some questions you can ask yourself as you are reading an article.

Did the Researcher Use the Correct Analysis?

Based on your knowledge of multivariate statistics, did the person seem to use the correct analysis? Figure 11.3 shows a flowchart that illustrates the relationship between many of the multivariate statistics we discussed in this chapter based on the number and type of dependent variables and independent variables. This chart can help you decide if the researcher used an appropriate analysis in the study. If there seems to be more than one possible analysis that could be used, did the researcher provide a rationale for why this particular analysis was used? If an infrequently used statistical analysis was performed, did the researcher provide a rationale for why it was chosen?

Are All the Important Variables Included?

The ability of the multivariate analysis to predict a phenomenon is only as good as the variables included in the analysis. If important variables are missing, then the correlation between the independent variables and the dependent variable will not be as strong as it could be. Therefore, ask yourself if the researcher has omitted key variables that you think may relate to the phenomenon. For example, if you were predicting marital satisfaction, then excluding conflict resolution skills would likely significantly lower the predictive ability of the analysis. Sometimes the exclusion of an important variable is an oversight on the part of the researcher. However, if the researcher is using a preexisting data set, then the omission of a key variable may simply be a limitation of the data set.

Was There a Discussion of Assumptions and Missing Data?

A researcher who knows how to correctly run a multivariate analysis will first confirm that the assumptions for the analysis have been met. For example, in Chapter 9 we discussed the importance of variables having a normal distribution. There are other assumptions that may also need to be met.[5] The key point is that you can have more faith in a researcher's analysis if it is made explicit that the assumptions underlying the

---

[5]Other examples include homoscedasticity (equal variance for a variable across the range of values for another variable), and the absence of either extremely high correlations (multicollinearity) or perfect correlations (singularity) between two or more independent variables.

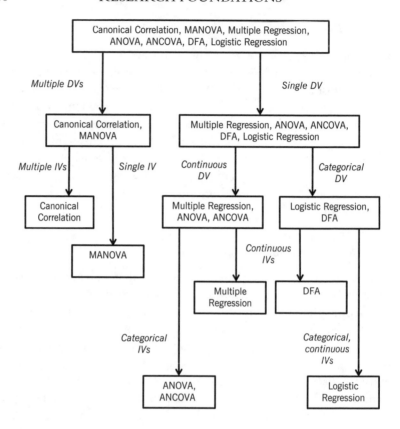

FIGURE 11.3. Multivariate flowchart diagram. *Note.* The covariate in an ANCOVA is continuous. DFA, discriminant function analysis.

analyses were tested. Unfortunately, most researchers do not make this explicit, but it is a notable strength if they do.

Researchers must often contend with another common problem, which is missing data. Missing data can occur if respondents fail to complete the survey, or if they skip over answering some questions. Again, ideally researchers will make explicit how they dealt with this problem, which gives you greater confidence in the analyses.[6]

---

[6]There are different strategies for dealing with missing data. In some cases, deleting all of the respondent's answers may be appropriate if there is too much missing data. If there is limited missing data, then the average score across all individuals can be substituted for a missing data point (called *mean substitution*). An alternative approach is to predict the missing value based on other information provided by the respondent.

Is the Sample Size Large Enough?

Multivariate analyses require a large enough sample size to avoid overfitting. Overfitting occurs when the ratio of cases to independent variables is not large enough, leading to an equation that has a stronger ability to predict than in real life. The ratio of cases to independent variables depends upon a number of factors. However, you should suspect overfitting if the sample size is small (less than 100–200) and includes several independent variables.

Clinical Application: Thinking in a Multivariate Way

You probably have not gone into the therapy room with multivariate statistics on your mind. However, the basic idea behind multivariate statistics has implications for how we can conceptualize our work. We need to ask ourselves, "Are we multivariate thinkers when we do therapy?" In other words, are we being attentive to the multiple factors that may contribute to a problem or outcome?

If you are accustomed to working with multiple family members, then it is probably natural for you to think in a multivariate way. Rather than focus just on an individual, you have likely been trained to see how multiple family members' actions can contribute to the creation or maintenance of a problem. However, our clients may not always think in a multivariate way. Clients may attribute the problem to a single person. In family work, for example, a child may be labeled as the identified patient by the parents.

Clients and therapists also need to avoid assuming that problems are caused by a single factor, because there may be multiple underlying causes. For example, Veronica breaks down into tears and tells the therapist how she recently discovered her husband, Lance, had an affair with her cousin Alyssa. Lance had dated Alyssa prior to the marriage, but Alyssa ended the relationship before Veronica and Lance became a couple. Veronica's explanation for why Lance had the affair with Alyssa was a simple one—Lance really loved Alyssa, but had settled for Veronica since Alyssa was not available. Through further assessment it became clear that the reasons for the affair did not fit Veronica's explanation, and that there were actually multiple factors that helped create it.

The affair began shortly after Veronica and Lance began to have problems. One night while having sex, Veronica's memories related to previous sexual abuse were triggered. Although she did not blame Lance for this, she was reluctant to engage in sexual intimacy because of the negative emotions this triggered. Unfortunately, Lance experienced this as rejection, and he began to withdraw. Because Lance had no close friends, he discussed his problem with one of the few people he felt comfortable confiding in, Alyssa. It was also discovered that Alyssa initiated the affair because she was angry with Veronica over a family conflict. Although Lance did not intend for the affair to happen, his loneliness and distress over his marital problems made him vulnerable to an affair. The couple was helped to see how the affair arose due to a complex set of factors.

Multivariate statistics such as MANOVA and canonical correlation also remind us that there may be multiple outcome variables that require our attention. As therapists, we may become focused on one particular outcome, while ignoring others. For example, McFarlane et al. (2003) described how early research on family-based treatments for treating schizophrenia focused on measuring relapse rates for schizophrenia (e.g., hospitalizations). However, many of the individuals struggling with schizophrenia discussed other quality of life issues that were of concern to them, such as employment or quality of social relationships. Research in this field is now evolving to include these outcomes as well. Couple therapists or researchers may focus exclusively on the marital or relationship outcomes, overlooking how the couple's relationship impacts the children. However, it may also be important to look at child outcomes when working with couples. For example, one study evaluated behavioral couples therapy for treating substance abuse included measures for evaluating child well-being, and discovered improved outcomes for children even though they were not directly included in the treatment (Kelley & Fals-Stewart, 2002).

PART II

Evidence-Based Practice

CHAPTER 12

What Is an Evidence–Based Approach?

Andrea looks at a new referral form from the school. Her future clients are Ralph (age 8), who has been diagnosed with autism, and Ralph's divorced, unemployed mother. They have been ordered to attend therapy after Ralph became aggressive at school. Andrea wonders if she is up to the task of helping Ralph and his mother. Her agency supervisor gave her the referral so he must think she is capable of helping them, but Andrea has never treated a child with autism before. Andrea is also a single, childless 24-year-old and she concedes that she knows little about the challenges the mother faces. In addition, Andrea's supervisor uses psychodynamic theory almost exclusively in Andrea's supervision. Andrea wonders how helpful psychodynamic ideas will be for her new case.

What might Andrea do next to help herself ask the right questions during her assessment? How can Andrea create a treatment plan that has the best chance of helping Ralph and his mother? How will Andrea make these decisions? Evidence-based practice is designed to help Andrea answer these questions.

Once Andrea learns some basic evidence-based skills, she can apply them to any new client situation she encounters. As with learning any new skill, Andrea will probably need to spend some time learning the basics of evidence-based practice. This process may require some extra time at the onset, but once Andrea becomes competent using the skills, she will be able to quickly find accurate, useful information that will help her make informed decisions about her clinical work. By using evidence-based practice she will be providing the best possible care available to her clients.

Evidence-based practice (EBP) is the integration of *best research evidence* with *clinical expertise* and *patient values* (Patterson, Miller, Carnes, & Wilson, 2004; Sackett, Straus, Richardson, Rosenberg, & Haynes, 2000). In recent years, an expanded definition included consideration of the *environmental and organizational context* as well (Council for Training in Evidence-Based Behavioral Practice, 2008). In essence, when you use EBP, you use research findings to guide your treatment decisions. EBP is about *using* research, not collecting data yourself.

You may want to ask yourself, "How do I currently make treatment decisions?" Common answers include:

"I was trained in a particular model or theory, so that is the one I use."

"People I respect (experts) use specific ideas, so I do too."

"I do not follow any one model. I just do whatever seems relevant in the moment."

These are all potentially useful rationales for making assessment and treatment decisions. But EBP posits that all of the work done by researchers on a specific problem or diagnosis is the best guide for clinical decision making, although it is not the only guide. We also recognize research findings may be difficult to apply in some instances. For example, treatment X may have strong evidence, but it may not be available in your community. However, research still can be an invaluable tool as you start making assessment and treatment decisions.

A BRIEF HISTORY —
OF EVIDENCE-BASED PRACTICE

EBP has its roots in the United States in the early 20th century and in the United Kingdom when Archibald Cochrane argued for funding health care that had empirical support (Spring, 2007). The principles of EBP were ultimately developed at McMaster University in Canada during the 1980s. A group of scholars wanted to discover improved methods for finding, evaluating, and applying clinical research (Patterson et. al, 2004). They had the ultimate goal of finding better ways of deciding what new information should be incorporated into their practices. In one early article, the founders of EBP said:

> [EBP] will help you translate the results of medical research into clinical practice. We've written them from the perspective of the busy clinician who wants to provide effective medical care but is sharply restricted in time for reading. . . . [EBP] is about using, not doing, research. It is designed to help provide our patients with care that is based on the best evidence currently available. (Oxman, Sackett, & Guyatt, 1993, p. 2093)

Since the eighties, many human service professions have adopted evidence-based principles including psychology, behavioral medicine, social work, education, and others. Also, employers, insurance agencies, and other stakeholders have begun to require that clinicians use EBP. A great deal of work has been done to gather evidence through research and to create user-friendly efficient ways for the busy clinician to locate the evidence. A prime example of this process is a government agency called the Agency for Healthcare Research and Quality (AHRQ) that created a center to gather evidence on healthcare topics (*www.ahrq.gov/clinic/epc*). Additionally, the AHRQ is funding Translating Research into Practice projects (TRIP-I, TRIP-II) that evaluate how effectively research-based approaches can be successfully implemented in applied settings (*www.ahrq.gov/research/trip2fac.htm*). Scholars emphasize the importance of recognizing the context in which the findings will be applied. The preferences of therapists and clients have been noted as important factors in making treatment decisions.

OVERVIEW OF THE EVIDENCE-BASED PRACTICE STEPS: THE FIVE A's

In a nutshell, EBP has five steps (Spring, Abrantes, Kreslake, & Hitchcock, 2007):

1. Converting the need for information into an answerable question.
2. Locating the best evidence to answer the question.
3. Critical appraisal of validity, impact, and applicability of research.
4. Integrating clinical appraisal with our clinical expertise, patient preferences, and clinical context.
5. Evaluating the effectiveness and efficiency of chosen treatments.

Scholars summarize this process with **five A's: Ask, Acquire, Appraise, Apply, and Analyze and adjust** (Spring et al., 2007). More information about each step will be explored in the following paragraphs, but memorizing the five A's is an easy way to remember the basic process. The subsequent chapters in this book will present more detailed information around each of the five A's.

In addition to what you will learn in this book, the Internet can also be a resource for learning more about EBP. For example, the Evidence-Based Behavioral Practice website (*www.ebbp.org/training.html*) has several training modules for learning about various aspects of EBP. The Columbia University School of Social Work also has a site that has multiple training modules on EBP (*www.columbia.edu/cu/musher/Website/Website/EBP_OnlineTraining.htm*). You can easily find other resources by doing a search with the keywords *evidence-based practice*.

Ask (Step 1): Create a Question That Can Be Answered by the Literature

This skill takes some practice. It is helpful to have familiarity with the research literature so that you can pick out keywords. Another useful skill that makes this process easier is learning how to narrow down your question. Your question needs to be narrow enough so that you are not overwhelmed by information that does not apply to you. However, it is still important to have your question be broad enough so that you will find results.

For example, Andrea might ask the following question: What treatments work for autism? In this question, her keyword is *autism*. If Andrea searches for *autism*, she will be overwhelmed with literature (unless she used a database of systematic reviews—more on this later). This is in an indication that her search is too broad. If she is reviewing the studies herself, she may become frustrated and overwhelmed with the amount of literature she has to sift through. Andrea might want to narrow her search by asking a more specific question. An example of a relevant specific question would be: What brief, family-based treatments work best for treating aggressive symptoms in a child with autism? In this question, she has narrowed her search by adding keywords including *brief, family based,* and *aggressive symptoms*. The addition of these keywords will narrow her search significantly. However, these words may make her search too narrow and significantly reduce the amount of articles recovered in her search.

Another challenge family therapists may encounter includes searching for nonmedical language and experiences. As stated earlier, evidence-based literature developed first in the medical field, so one will still find a bias for biomedical language in the databases. Additionally, many research articles have difficulty capturing psychosocial concepts. Andrea might find a great deal of literature on treating autism but find nothing if she asks the following question: How does divorce affect an autistic child?

Andrea would quickly realize in her search of the literature that there is more empirical literature on autism than there is on divorce. Perhaps Andrea learns that Ralph's aggressive symptoms became more pronounced immediately after Ralph's father left him and his mother. She believes there is a link between the parent's divorce and Ralph's aggression, but she will have trouble finding that link clearly demonstrated in the literature. Andrea will have to use her clinical judgment and expertise to extrapolate from the research she finds, while also considering Ralph's behaviors and his mother's preferences as she moves forward. The "art" of therapy remains extremely relevant in EBP.

During assessment Andrea might learn about other factors that will influence her clinical course of treatment. For example, Andrea might discover that Ralph's mother has been clinically depressed since Ralph's father left. Additionally, she might also learn that Ralph has Tourette syndrome and lived with his grandmother until he was 5 years old. As Andrea learns more about Ralph's situation, she realizes she has several questions and could conduct several searches. Her questions might include:

- How does maternal depression affect a child's development?
- What is the relationship between Tourette syndrome and autism?
- How do changes in home environment affect aggressive behavior in children, especially autistic children?

Each of these questions reflects one part of a complex case. It is unlikely Andrea will find studies or answers that combine all of these client characteristics. Andrea will need to prioritize her clinical questions and treatment goals. As Andrea finds several studies addressing different aspects of Ralph's case, she will have to use her clinical judgment to put the puzzle of findings together into a coherent whole treatment plan. This skill takes practice, familiarity with the literature, and clinical acumen.

Andrea may conduct an EBP search on one topic as a starting point and learn that treatment X has the most empirical support for that problem. However, she may not be familiar with treatment X and no one in her office or her community has expertise delivering treatment X. Andrea faces several different treatment decisions in this situation, but at least she has a foundation of knowledge about effective treatments. Andrea always has the option to keep searching. She may refine her search based on the resources that exist in her setting.

Acquire (Step 2): Locate the Best Evidence to Answer the Question

As clearly evident above, being able to locate research to answer your question is an important skill set. Being able to effectively and efficiently locate research pertinent to your questions requires knowledge of different databases. Some databases contain articles on specific research studies, while other databases, such as the Cochrane Library, specialize in providing reviews of the research in different areas. It is also important that you have effective strategies for searching within databases to locate salient articles or reviews. The next chapter will address both of these elements when conducting a search.

There are two important considerations affecting how you carry out step two that are seldom mentioned in the evidence-based literature: time and money, or, in other words, the cost of the databases and the "cost" of your own professional time. Most therapists fondly remember their days in graduate school when they had the luxury of spending hours exploring their intellectual interests by browsing scholarly literature, but now as busy professionals, "time is money." Often in clinical work, the time to search the literature is usurped by productivity demands, usually measured in terms of patient contact hours.

Fortunately, as stated above, there are databases (e.g., Cochrane Library) that contain reviews of the research that do most of the work for the therapist in terms of locating and summarizing the research. If you do have access to them, these databases save considerable time. Some of these databases not only summarize findings from individual research studies but also make specific recommendations based on the data. These recommendations might even be graded on the strength or power of the research supporting that particular recommendation. For example, behavioral family therapy might have a strong recommendation as a treatment option for a family member with attention-deficit/

hyperactivity disorder. Instead of reviewing and evaluating multiple studies to create a treatment plan yourself, you are able to turn to one credible source such as the Cochrane Library and simply read the treatment recommendations.

Unfortunately, even if a therapist has time to research her client's mental health struggles, she might not have easy or free access to the databases necessary to do the search. The ability to use a university or community college library makes it feasible to access multiple databases. Some research can also be found through the Internet by using search engines like Google Scholar or PubMed, although the clinician may need to pay to access the article from the publisher. Membership in professional organizations may allow therapists to access some databases. For example, members of the California Association of Marriage and Family Therapists have access to EBSCO*host*, permitting them to search a large database with psychotherapy research.

Appraise (Step 3): Evaluate the Literature

While many busy clinicians bypass this step by relying on summaries that review and evaluate the existing research on a topic, it is still a good idea to possess the skills necessary to evaluate the primary sources. There may be times when you have the time and motivation to look at the original research. For example, you might want to know how closely the clients who received the study treatment match your current client. You might realize that different statistical analyzes produce different results and you might want to understand exactly how the analyses were done in a particular study. There may even be some situations where there is not enough literature for reviews to exist. In some rare cases, your client's problems may not even be identified in the literature. For example, until recently there was little empirical literature on sexual addiction even though therapists were beginning to see an increasing number of clients struggling with sexual addiction. Thus, sometimes the best you can do is to evaluate the one or two existing studies yourself.

Usually, Step 3 refers to evaluating the quantitative methods and research design of studies related to your client's problems, but you can also extend the scope of Step 3 by including literature that is qualitative in nature. You may find ideas in a variety of research designs that may be helpful with your particular clinical scenario. The first half of this book provides the information and skills you need to evaluate a variety of research designs. Chapter 14 will also provide more information on how to read and evaluate research studies, as well as how to evaluate systematic reviews.

An increasingly common scenario occurs when your client brings you information that he or she found on the Internet about their problem, or perhaps your client may have talked to a friend who recommends a particular treatment. This could be a good sign of your client's motivation to change. In these situations, your client has already started Steps 1 and 2. This may require that you evaluate the level of empirical support for this particular treatment. Together, you could explore the literature your client found and move on together to Steps 4 and 5.

Apply (Step 4): Integrate Clinical Appraisal with Our Clinical Expertise, Client Preferences, and Context

Step 4 encourages therapists to use their personal expertise and client preferences in deciding how to best help their clients. The founders of EBP state that clinical expertise refers to a therapist's unique skills and experiences, while client preferences includes the values, concerns, and expectations that clients bring to the clinical encounter (Sackett et. al., 2000). Some therapists might be reluctant to use evidence-based skills because they worry that it will lead to a "cookbook" approach to treatment, especially as **manualized treatments** become increasingly common. They worry that EBP will invade the therapeutic relationship and the caring and concern that is at the heart of good therapy will be subsumed by rote protocols.

Step 4 suggests these fears need not materialize. Information gleaned from evidence-based resources is at best a guide. The reductionist quality of some empirical studies where there may be only two or three variables that are thoroughly explored are not meant to replace the human wisdom or the empathic attunement that the therapist and client can share.

Chapter 15 will address how therapists can translate research findings into clinical practice, including some of the potential challenges that may be encountered. For example, a therapist knows that a particular treatment has ameliorated similar problems for similar clients (therapeutic effectiveness). The therapist might also consider the "efficiency" of the treatment. Perhaps the treatment is too costly, takes too long, or the therapist might not be familiar with the treatment and might consider referring the client to a colleague who does know about a specific treatment protocol.

One potential way therapists can incorporate research into their clinical work is to learn and use models that have empirical support for their effectiveness. Chapter 16 will discuss various models from the family therapy literature that therapists can use to address problems they frequently encounter in practice.

In Step 4, the therapist and client might review the findings from EBP sources and decide what they want to consider in their treatment process. In addition, they might explore what alterations they might make in the treatment protocols to optimize the chance of the treatment working in a specific setting. Talking about evidence-based treatment options with your client may strengthen the therapeutic relationship because your client has the opportunity to gain respect for your expertise and recognizes the care and thought you are putting into her care. Chapter 17 will explore in more detail how therapists and clients can work together to make shared decisions on how to apply EBP to treatment.

Analyze and Adjust (Step 5): Evaluate the Effectiveness and Efficiency of the Chosen Treatment

Often assessment and treatment are continuous, and at times, interchangeable in therapy. For example, focusing attention on a mental health problem by conducting a thorough assessment can simultaneously be an intervention (Williams, Edwards, Patterson, & Chamow, 2011). During the assessment, the client may realize the seriousness of a problem that they may have been ignoring and decide they are ready to make some changes.

From the first appointment, both the therapist and client continuously ask themselves, "Is what we are doing helping?" "Is the client improving?" Chapter 18 will explore ways therapists can evaluate how therapy is going. Practical and easily implemented tools for monitoring client progress and the client–therapist alliance will be introduced. Using these tools to evaluate therapy increases the likelihood that therapy will be effective.

Evaluation is usually not a one-time event. Instead, the therapist must continually adjust the treatment to new circumstances or challenges. For example, Andrea might know that some behavioral treatments might help Ralph become less aggressive, but she soon learns that Ralph's mother is so overwhelmed that she is unable to systematically and consistently deliver the behavioral treatment at home. Thus, Andrea might amend the recommended treatment protocol so that it fits the challenging life circumstances that Ralph and his mother face each day.

CONCLUSION

When the authors teach basic principles of EBP, students often raise several concerns. Questions they raise include:

> "What should I do if I do not know the most effective keywords to conduct a search?"
>
> "What if I do not know much about the databases used in an EBP search?"
>
> "What should I do if I discover that I do not know how to deliver an evidence-based treatment?"
>
> "How do I integrate evidence-based treatments for different problems?"
>
> "What should I do if I do not have time to conduct an EBP search on all of my clients' diagnoses and problems?"

These are all normal concerns for a therapist trying to apply research findings to their clinical work. During their coursework, students often wonder about the application of the knowledge they learn in their research classes to their clinical work. Ideally, clinical supervisors teach EBP skills alongside teaching clinical skills. Also, as students become more familiar with the evidence-based literature, they become more efficient and self-confident. Most therapists remember when they were first learning how to play a sport, cook a meal, or learn any new skill. They practiced the skills over and over. Practicing skills was often less satisfying and rewarding than eventually seeing the results of the hours of training, such as a big win or a great meal. Learning evidence-based skills might be a similar experience, but over time the five steps can become second nature. Therapists can learn to quickly and efficiently review literature and decide what matches their unique setting. They can also feel confident knowing that they are bringing all of the resources of scientific inquiry to the challenges their clients face.

CHAPTER 13

Ask and Acquire

Creating Questions and Conducting a Search

Once one has decided to use evidence-based skills in clinical work, one has to learn the skills in order to do so. In the previous chapter we introduced you to the five A's: Ask, Acquire, Appraise, Apply, and Analyze and adjust. This chapter will focus on the first two A's, Ask and Acquire. One must be able to learn the essential ability to ask the right question(s) and to find relevant information. These two processes are linked because the type of questions you ask may impact what type of sources you look for and where you might find them. Thus, one has to be familiar with the types of resources that are available to you when performing a search. We will also discuss how to expand or narrow one's search when trying to identify research to answer your questions.

DEFINING THE PURPOSE OF THE SEARCH

What do you hope to learn by doing a search? This is an important question because it will define what you look for and where you might find the answer. Research can be used to answer various types of questions. For example, you may want to search for information about how to treat a specific family problem or an individual mental disorder. While your questions will usually focus on a search for treatment recommendations, you might at times have other types of questions.

Gibbs (2003) identifies five types of questions: effectiveness, prevention, risk/prognosis, assessment, and description. Each question type suggests different purposes behind the search. An example of each type of question is listed below:

- Is neurofeedback effective (effectiveness)?
- How can families prevent teenagers from abusing alcohol (prevention)?
- Will shy children have social phobia when they grow up (risk)?
- How can you tell when a client with grief has developed depression that needs to be treated (assessment)?
- What are the effects of long-term child abuse (description)?

More specific questions within each of these domains can be created by using questions that begin with W words—*who, what, where, when,* or *why* (Walker, 2007). For example, the following questions might be asked when searching for treatment recommendations:

- *Who* is most (or least) likely to benefit from treatment Y?
- *What* treatments are effective for treating condition X?
- *What* is the success rate if treatment Y is used to treat condition X or problem Z?
- *What* are the most important elements (active ingredients) to treatment Y?
- *Where* can treatment Y be effectively delivered (e.g., home, therapy office, inpatient)?
- *When* is treatment W a better option than treatment Y?
- *Why* do clients drop out of treatment Y?

Questions that follow the **PICO** format—that is, **P**atient group or population, **I**ntervention, **C**omparison group, and **O**utcome measures—can also be used to formulate more specific questions for treatment-oriented inquiries. Examples of PICO questions might include:

- What patient groups has the treatment been shown to be effective for?
- What intervention or treatment is most effective for treating condition X?

- What comparison group has the treatment been demonstrated to be more effective than (e.g., no treatment control, treatment as usual)?
- What outcome measures have been used to evaluate the effectiveness of the treatment?

The W words can also be used to help construct helpful questions in other domains too. Consider the following examples:

- *Who* is most likely to benefit from preventative treatment Y (prevention)?
- *Who* is most likely to seek out preventative treatment Y (prevention)?
- *What* is the effectiveness of treatment Y in preventing problem Z (prevention)?
- *When* is treatment Y most effectively delivered to prevent problem Z (prevention)?
- *Who* is most likely to develop condition X or problem Z (risk)?
- *What* factors predict condition X or problem Z (risk)?
- *What* factors differentiate the diagnosis between conditions X and V (assessment)?
- *What* are reliable and valid instruments for measuring condition X (assessment)?
- *What* do individuals who have condition X normally experience (description)?
- *What* are the biggest challenges clients with condition X must face (description)?
- *What* are common strategies clients use successfully to cope with condition X or problem Z (description)?

In clinical practice, therapists doing searches generally seek guidance on what to do next to help their clients. For example, a therapist that has limited knowledge about a problem that the family is presenting may initially do a search to gain general information about the problem (e.g., assessment, description, risk/prognosis). After this phase, direct treatment guidelines are probably what therapists will seek when doing an evidence-based search. In this way, evidence-based searches are "electronic supervisors"—they nudge the therapist to the most appropriate treatments.

FRAMING THE QUESTION USING KEYWORDS

Learning how to frame your question is one of the most important skills you need for evidence-based work. Framing the question properly will help you get the answer you need and determine good follow-up questions. Using keywords is an important element in effectively framing questions.

During graduate school, therapists will have to become familiar with using keywords to do library searches. The same skills are needed for evidence-based searches. You have to be able to condense your questions or concerns into a question that can be answered by the literature. This skill takes practice and familiarity with the evidence-based resources. In general, common words from medical literature or the *Diagnostic and Statistical Manual of Mental Disorders* (American Psychiatric Association, 2013) are easier to find than words from less common theoretical models. Thus, you will find literature and recommendations on treating anorexia nervosa, but less on enmeshed families or boundaries, even though all three terms might apply to your client family.

Some databases, such as PsycINFO and PubMed, offer an aid to using keywords called a *thesaurus search*. PsycINFO has over 8,000 terms in its thesaurus. As you become more familiar with different sources, you will also learn which sites use a thesaurus for a controlled vocabulary search and which ones leave it up to the searcher to decide the keywords.

Another strategy for identifying keywords is to examine the references of articles you have located in your initial search. By inspecting the titles of publications cited within these articles, you may be able to find additional keywords for expanding your search. For example, if you are interested in studying religious differences among couples, you might discover that some researchers (particularly those in the family studies field) use the term *religious heterogamy*. However, this is not a keyword that would immediately come to mind for most therapists.

Sometimes your questions may involve multiple ideas. Terms such as *and*, *or*, and *not* can be used to limit or expand your search (Collins & Ladd, 2007). Also, most sources use very specific keywords. For example, you may be interested in how bullying affects depressed teens. You might do a search containing the words *bullies*, *bully*, *bullying*. However, on many sites an asterisk allows you to search all three words simultaneously by starting out with the root word and then using the asterisk at the end, such as *bull**.

If you need extra help with the search process, there are quick guides available to assist you. One example of this is the Evidence Based Medicine Tool Kit (*www.ebm.med.ualberta.ca*) from the University of Alberta, which also includes worksheets designed to help you evaluate sources (Buckingham, Fisher, & Saunders, 2012).

DIFFERENT TYPES OF SOURCES

Figure 13.1 illustrates the types of sources you could possibly use to answer your questions (Collins & Ladd, 2007; Davidson, Trudeau, Ockene, Orleans, & Kaplan, 2004; Patterson et al., 2004). Sources can be categorized as either primary or secondary. **Primary sources** are the original research studies. Typically, research is published in the form of journal articles, although they can also be found in other forms such as dissertations, technical reports, or conference proceedings.

Secondary sources synthesize the research from primary sources. They can take several forms, including traditional literature reviews, sys-

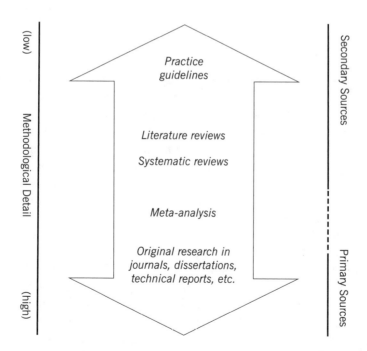

FIGURE 13.1. Primary and secondary resources.

tematic reviews, and practice guidelines. **Systematic reviews** use a rigorous approach to select, locate, evaluate, and synthesize research studies to answer specific questions. Evaluating systematic reviews is discussed in Chapter 14. **Practice guidelines** provide treatment recommendations and summaries formed from evidence-based literature. These may be based upon systematic reviews, expert consensus, or other means. Secondary sources can be found in many different places including journal articles, textbooks, policy papers, or on websites.

Meta-analysis (see Chapter 7) shares characteristics of both primary and secondary sources. Because it is original research, meta-analysis is like a primary source. However, it empirically synthesizes the results from multiple studies, so it is similar to secondary sources in this regard.

One of the advantages of using secondary resources is that someone else has taken the time and energy to locate and synthesize the research for you. This can save you considerable time over locating and reviewing each of the studies yourself. In some cases, the secondary sources may even evaluate the quality of the research, saving you further time and effort. Thus different sites may give both a summary recommendation and an evaluation of how strong the research is that supports the recommendation.

To ensure the integrity of the recommendations, some groups use experts and other groups to carefully conduct systematic reviews. The site may have specific standards for inclusion because the editors of the site recognize that there is a broad range in the quality of evidence, with the randomized clinical trial being the gold standard of evidence. For example, the American Psychological Association developed task forces and very specific criteria for evaluating treatments so clinicians would know how much confidence they could place in a treatment. Government agencies, professional associations, governing boards, and other groups set their own guidelines for inclusion in evidence-based reviews. Some groups require randomized clinical trials and treatment manuals and other groups do not.

Instead of an all or nothing approach, some groups "grade" the quality of the evidence with adjectives such as "strong" or with letter grades such as "A, B, or C." Unfortunately, there is no universal consensus on what constitutes an evidence-based or universal evaluation system, especially in mental health. However, an increasing number of EBP groups are using information from the GRADE working group (*www.gradeworkinggroup.org*). This group of scholars started working together in 2000 and has developed a popular approach to grading quality of evidence and strength of recommendations. As you become familiar with a few sources, you will simultaneously become familiar with their evaluation systems.

KNOWING WHERE TO LOOK

Knowing where to look for primary and secondary sources is another important skill used in EBP. Table 13.1 lists several important databases clinicians may want to use. The list is not comprehensive but includes many of the most well-known evidence-based sources.

PsycINFO and EBSCO*host* are particularly good databases for searching for primary sources within the mental health field. Although both have a subscription fee, they can be frequently accessed through many university and community colleges. PubMed offers free access to the Medline database, which is excellent for locating primary sources within the medical field. HighWire is another database that can be used for free to locate primary research in the medical, science, or social sciences. In some cases, articles located through PubMed or HighWire can be downloaded for free, while others may require a fee to download. The above sites can also be searched for meta-analyses and secondary sources (e.g., literature reviews, systematic reviews).

Some of the databases specialize in providing literature reviews or systematic reviews. Examples of these databases include the Cochrane Database of Systematic Reviews, UpToDate, and the Campbell Collaboration. Other sources provide practice guidelines based on research, but do not offer detailed descriptions of the research. For example, the American Psychological Association provides an overview and treatment recommendations for a number of topics.

You can also search for research through search engines on the Internet like Google or GoogleScholar (*http://scholar.google.com*). You might also consider using meta-search engines that search several search engines at the same time and combines all of the results. For example, *dogpile.com* will search Google, Yahoo, Bing, and Yandex all at once.

Which type of source and database you use will depend upon a number of factors. One factor that it will depend upon is the nature of your clinical questions. For example, it may be easier to locate reviews that summarize the outcome research. The databases you search may also change as your questions evolve. A search usually begins with general questions and then transitions to a search for specific recommendations.

TABLE 13.1. Where to Look for Primary and Secondary Information (Alphabetical)

Agency for Healthcare Research and Quality's HCUP
http://hcupnet.ahrq.gov

AHRQ is a federal agency that advances EBP in a number of ways. One of its functions is to support the Healthcare Cost and Utilization Project (HCUP), a free database of health statistics.

Agency for Healthcare Research and Quality's National Guideline Clearinghouse
http://guideline.gov/index.aspx

In addition to HCUP, AHRQ also provides free access to the National Guidelines Clearinghouse, a database of treatment guidelines and expert commentaries on various diagnoses.

American Psychiatric Association Practice Guidelines
www.psych.org/practice/clinical-practice-guidelines

This website includes evidence-based recommendations for the assessment and treatment of adult psychiatric disorders. These guidelines are free and include information for locating child guidelines.

American Psychological Association Guidelines
www.apa.org/practice/guidelines/index.aspx

This website includes several topics that each come with an overview of the literature as well as treatment recommendations. These guidelines are free and do not require membership.

California Evidence-Based Clearinghouse for Child Welfare
www.cebc4cw.org

This website describes a variety of programs aimed at promoting child welfare in different areas, including treating mental illness. In addition to describing each program, the site rates the level of research support for each program. Access to this website is free.

Campbell Collaboration
www.campbellcollaboration.org

The Campbell Collaboration publishes systematic reviews in the areas of education, crime and justice, and social welfare. Access to this website is free.

Center for EBM
http://ktclearinghouse.ca/cebm

This website serves as a guide for those seeking evidence. It includes educational tools, such as glossaries and search guides, for those that are new to evidence-based medicine. It also includes a list of evidence-based resources. Access to this website is free.

Cochrane Database of Systematic Reviews
www.thecochranelibrary.com/view/0/index.html

The Cochrane Collaboration is a group of providers, patients, advocates, and policy makers. One of the functions of this group is to publish *Cochrane Reviews*, which are systematic reviews of medical literature. Some people are eligible for free access to these reviews while others need to pay for access. Check the website to see if you are eligible for free access.

EBSCO*host*
http://search.ebscohost.com

EBSCO*host* is a system that includes access to several different databases, resulting in the ability to cast a broader search that includes several different types of sources. Access to EBSCO*host* requires a paid subscription.

Embase
www.embase.com

Embase is a database that includes all of Medline as well as several other sources. It covers biomedical peer-reviewed journals as well as conferences and articles-in-press. Embase requires a paid subscription.

Evidence-Based Mental Health
http://ebmh.bmj.com

This is a journal that includes the key details from articles published in a wide variety of other biomedical journals. Access to this journal requires a paid subscription.

HighWire
http://highwire.stanford.edu

HighWire is a database hosted by Stanford that contains publications from journals in medicine, science, and social science. Searching the database is free, and includes links to free full-text for some articles depending upon the journal from which they come.

MedLine
www.nlm.nih.gov/pubs/factsheets/medline.html

MedLine is a database from the U.S. National Library of Medicine containing publications from over 5,600 different journals. Searching the database is free, but most full-text articles require a fee to access.

PsycINFO
www.apa.org/pubs/databases/psycinfo/index.aspx

PsycINFO is the American Psychological Association's database of peer-reviewed articles, books, and dissertations. Searching PsycINFO requires a paid subscription.

PubMed
www.ncbi.nlm.nih.gov/pubmed

PubMed is a database from the U.S. National Library of Medicine that includes all of MedLine as well as some other journals. Searching the database is free and includes links to free full-text articles for some articles depending on which journal they come from.

TRIP
www.tripdatabase.com

This is a database that includes several journals and allows clinicians to locate high-quality research quickly. Searching TRIP is free, but not all of the articles are available in full text for free.

UpToDate
www.uptodate.com

UpToDate is a database of literature reviews written by experts in various fields. Full access requires a paid subscription.

Eventually, one might have a more detailed question that can only be answered using primary source data. For example, a family therapist may search UpToDate to learn basic information about eating disorders. The therapist may then decide to compare behavioral family therapy versus medication and do a search on Cochrane. The therapist may learn that behavioral family therapy is especially effective with younger patients and their families, but he or she may still wonder if the ethnicity of the family influences the effectiveness of the treatment. Thus, the therapist may further search using PubMed for specific questions about the influence of ethnicity on the effectiveness of the treatment.

The amount of time you have to invest in a search is another factor that may influence which databases you use. When physicians initially formulated evidence-based ideas in Canada during the 1980s, scholars thought the new paradigm would revolutionize how medicine was practiced (Sackett, Haynes, Tugwell, & Guyatt, 1991). In reality, physicians frequently do not use evidence-based information at every patient visit and patients often do not understand the physician's evidence-based recommendations. Perhaps the single most important reason healthcare providers fail to use evidence-based principles is their sense of limited time and competing demands. The same dilemmas occur in psychotherapy practices. In addition, searching the literature is often unreimbursed time and many therapists measure their "productivity" on how many client contacts they have per day. Thus, at the beginning of your search, you might decide how much time you have to spend searching.

If you have limited time, you might instead simply seek treatment recommendations such as those sponsored by the American Psychiatric Association (*www.psych.org/practice/clinical-practice-guidelines*) or the American Psychological Association (*www.div12.org/PsychologicalTreatments*). Or as an alternative, if your site has purchased a resource such as UpToDate, then you might take 10 minutes between clients to do a quick search. However, if there is not enough solid research on your question, you may find that the topic is not included in a list of treatment/practice guidelines or reviews. You then may have to do more research to find the relevant information that exists on your topic.

Your own knowledge base also influences the amount of time it takes you to do a search. If you have a client with a problem or diagnosis that you have never treated before, you first want to obtain some general knowledge about the problem. In essence, you need to know enough about the problem to know what the possible treatment options are. Therefore, you might search a database like UpToDate or EBSCO*host* first before researching specific treatment options. Once you have obtained some basic information, you are able to do more detailed searches that compare treatment options. If you are short on time, you might go immediately to databases that contain reviews of the research (e.g., Cochrane) that have already synthesized and evaluated the research. Otherwise, you can search for information yourself on databases that simply present the research with no evaluation of research quality.

Finally, another factor that may influence where you search is the databases to which you have access. Clinics or professional organizations are more likely to purchase subscriptions for their employees. Universities usually have paid subscriptions that have been purchased for the library. Individual clinicians in private practice are often unable to afford the yearly paid subscription fees, although they may have some access to some journals through professional organizations.

EXPANDING, NARROWING, AND ENDING YOUR SEARCH

When you are searching through the literature for information, you may have difficulty finding enough research to answer your question. Conversely, you may encounter too much material in your search. Therefore, we will discuss in this section how to expand or narrow your search as necessary. Finally, we will discuss how you know when it is time to end your search.

Expanding and Narrowing Your Search

Different strategies can be used to expand your search. As discussed earlier, making sure that you are using the appropriate keywords is important. If you have difficulty finding research in one database, you could try doing a search in a different database. For example, you may be able to find some research on treating mental health disorders in a medical database (e.g., PubMed, Medline) that you may not find in psychological database like PsycINFO.

If you are able to find some articles that are relevant to your questions, then you can often use citations to expand your search. By checking the reference list of these articles, you may be able to find previous research that addresses your questions. Locating these articles and inspecting their reference lists may lead you to other studies, creating a snowball effect. This strategy, however, will only lead you to older research than the original articles. So, this works best if you have been able to locate a very recent study.

However, some databases indicate which other articles have cited the research that you have found. Thus, you may be able to expand your search to more recent research on the topic, which may lead you to other studies as well. To search the "web of knowledge" (researchers who are writing about a shared topic), you can use citation databases such as Thomson Reuters Web of Knowledge (*www.thomsonreuters.com/web-of-knowledge*) or Scopus (*www.info.sciverse.com/scopus*), or other databases like PsycINFO or Google Scholar that show you who has cited a particular article.

At times, you might also want to limit your search by adjusting your search criteria based on range of dates, type of publication (e.g., peer review), methodology, age of the population, and others factors. For example, you might limit your search to articles published in the past 10 years in peer-reviewed journals. Or, you could limit your search based on methodology to outcome studies or meta-analyses.

You can also limit your search by being more specific in the questions that you ask. For example, imagine you are working with a couple in therapy who is experiencing marital difficulties. The wife also has depression. If you did a search for articles in PsycINFO in which couple therapy appeared in the title, you would locate 1,655 articles. However, if you limited your search to articles that had both couple therapy and depression in the title, then you would narrow the number of articles down to 35.

Many of the more popular databases offer instructions or tutorials on their websites on how to most effectively conduct a search using their database. For example, PsycINFO has a Search Help and Training Center (*www.apa.org/pubs/databases/training/index.aspx*) that offers a variety of tools to help you become more skilled in PsycINFO. PubMed also offers a variety of resources for learning how to use the PubMed database (*www.nlm.nih.gov/bsd/disted/pubmed.html*). You can also find additional resources for conducting searches on EBP sites. For example, Module 2 of the EBBP website (Collins & Ladd, 2007) offers videos on searching the Cochrane Library, PubMed, and PsycINFO (see Appendix III for the specific links).

Deciding When to Stop

How will you know when you have completed your search and derived all of the critical information you may need in order to help your clients? There is no easy answer to this question and often may be determined by mundane forces, such as time limits and competing demands. However, metasearch engines such as TRIP (see Table 13.1) offer a rapid means to locate the best information. You could still continue your inquiry by doing a traditional search of nonempirical literature or other sources such as newsletters or websites. At times, treatment options are excluded not because the treatment will not work, but because the effectiveness of the treatment has not been evaluated through research. Ultimately, it is up to you to decide when you have acquired enough information in order to plan the next steps of your clients' treatments.

CONCLUSION

Over time you will develop the skills necessary to ask relevant, answerable questions. You will learn to prioritize your questions, which is an important skill if you have limited time and energy. Distinguishing between different types of questions (effectiveness, prevention, etc.) will become second nature. You will also become more knowledgeable on where to look for sources, including how to effectively search within various databases. Once you have located research, you can turn to evaluating its quality, which is the focus of our next chapter.

CHAPTER 14

Appraise

Reading and Evaluating
Research Articles and Systematic Reviews

In this chapter we discuss how to read and evaluate articles on single studies and systematic reviews that summarize multiple studies within an area. Articles of single studies can be important in answering clincial questions in a variety of ways. If you have a clinical question that is rather specific in nature, an individual study may offer an answer that is more relevant than a systematic review, which tends to look at broader questions. For example, you might be able to find a study that evaluates the effectiveness of a treatment with a specific population, whereas a meta-analysis or systematic review will likely examine the effectiveness of the treatment across a broader spectrum of individuals. In addition, you may have no alternative but to use single studies if no meta-analyses or systematic reviews are available because the existing research is limited.

However, systematic reviews can be quite helpful if they are available. Systematic reviews summarize the important research in one article, saving you considerable time in locating research articles. Authors of systematic reviews also do the job of synthesizing the information from numerous studies, which can be a challenge if there is a large number of studies. Thus, systematic reviews can be an efficient way to use research to inform your clinical work. Another advantage of systematic reviews is that the findings are based on multiple studies. Therefore, you often have greater confidence in the conclusions drawn from systematic reviews. In contrast, you may need to be more tentative applying your findings based on the results of a single research study.

READING A SINGLE RESEARCH STUDY

Journal articles on single research studies typically follow a set structure. In this section, we will describe the purpose of each section. We will also discuss possible short cuts one can take in reading a research study, including the potential tradeoffs in doing so. Ultimately, how you read a particular study will depend upon the purpose of your inquiry and what questions you are trying to answer. For example, if you want to identify key themes across multiple studies, then you may be able to quickly skim through several articles without reading them in their entirety. However, if you want to apply the findings from a specific study to a clinical case, then you will want to carefully read the entire article to determine the level of confidence you can place in the findings.

Abstract

The abstract is a brief summary of the research that usually does not exceed 150 words. Reading the abstract often gives you enough information to decide if the study is applicable to your question and is worth reading. However, the abstract typically does not give you enough information regarding the results and their implications. It also does not provide you the details you need to evaluate the quality or rigor of a study.

However, if you are simply trying to get a big picture view of the research in a particular area, reading the abstracts of several articles may give you sufficient information to identify the key themes. For example, if you are unfamiliar with a particular issue, reading outcome studies within that area may help you identify one or two approaches that seem to be commonly used. This, in turn, may lead you to learn more about those approaches.

Literature Review

The literature review is intended to give you a context for the study by summarizing the existing research on the topic and how it informs the current study. Researchers often conclude the literature review with the research questions the study will address, which should ideally flow from the discussion of the literature.

A good literature review will have several qualities. Most importantly, the literature review should build a strong case as to why the study is needed or important. Researchers often do this by identifying where there are gaps or limitations in the existing research and how the current study will address them. Ideally, a literature review should critique rather than simply summarize the existing research. In addition, a good literature review will include the most current research on the topic, yet be selective in choosing the most relevant studies, especially if there is an extensive amount of research on the topic. Finally, the purpose of the study, along with the research questions, should be clearly articulated.

Reading the literature review can help you understand how the current study fits into the existing research. It also aids you in identifying other studies that may be relevant to your question. If you skip reading the literature review, we strongly recommend you at least skim it to identify the purpose and research questions because the study will be organized around them.

Methods

Every research study should have a section that describes the methodology used to conduct the study. This has two purposes. First, it allows the reader to evaluate the rigor of the study, which helps you determine how much confidence to place in the findings. Second, it provides other researchers the information they need to replicate the study.

The methods section should make explicit what type of design was used (e.g., survey, experiment, content analysis, qualitative interviews), as well as the procedures that were followed. It should also describe how study participants were obtained (e.g., sampling approach), along with a summary of the sample's demographics. The methods section also needs to articulate how key variables were measured, including information on the reliability and validity of key measures.

Some individuals simply skip this section because they find the information difficult to understand. We hope you will be more comfortable and confident evaluating this section after reading this book. Reading the methods section allows you to directly evaluate the quality of the study. Otherwise, you will have to rely on indirect indicators of quality, which are much less reliable.

Results

The results section provides a detailed discussion of the findings from the study. Quantitative studies will summarize the results from the statistical analyses. Qualitative studies will present the analytical framework derived from the analysis, including quotes and descriptions to support the framework.

Results sections can sometimes be dense and somewhat difficult to read, particularly if there are a large number of statistical analyses. Therefore, individuals may be tempted to skip reading this section and rely on the discussion for an overview of the results. Again, our hope is that reading the results section will be less intimidating given the knowledge you have gained from this book. In some cases, skimming the results section may be a viable short cut, particularly if you are simply looking for themes across studies. However, there are two potential dangers in not carefully reading the results section. First, you risk missing important details about the findings that might get overlooked in the discussion. Second, skipping this section will make it difficult for you to identify conclusions in the discussion that are not warranted based on the results. For example, one of us recently reviewed a journal manuscript where the author concluded certain variables were important to understanding a phenomenon, yet some of these variables were never included in the analyses.

Discussion

The discussion section provides the researcher the opportunity to summarize the key results and speculate as to why certain results were found, especially if they were different from what was expected. The discussion is also the place where the researcher should articulate the key limitations of the study, as well as potential directions for future research. Ideally, the author will address the significance of the findings, including potential clinical or policy implications. Stronger studies will address both clinical and statistical significance when discussing the findings.

As we stated above, some individuals skip the methods and results sections and only read the discussion. However, if you don't read these sections, then you may be less likely to identify if the researcher has overstated the conclusions that can be drawn from the results.

References

Many individuals do not read the reference list. However, the reference list can help you locate other sources cited in the article that you might be interested in reading. In addition, as noted in the previous chapter, looking at the titles in the reference list might aid you in identifying keywords you can use to expand your search.

EVALUATING THE QUALITY OF A STUDY

It is important that you be able to evaluate the quality of a study by assessing its strengths and limitations. This determines the level of confidence you can place in the findings. Obviously, you will have more confidence in a study that uses a rigorous methodology compared to one with serious flaws.

When evaluating a study, it is important to recognize that no study will be perfect. Every study will have some limitations. However, some studies contain fatal flaws that undermine their credibility. As you gain more experience reading studies, it will become easier for you to distinguish the stronger studies from the weaker ones. Learning to read and evaluate a study is a skill that improves with practice.

The best manner for evaluating the quality of a study is to read the entire article, especially the methods section. Using the concepts we have discussed in the first half of the book, you have the necessary knowledge and skills to identify the key strengths and limitations of a study. This does not mean you won't encounter information with which you are unfamiliar, but you will have sufficient knowledge to know if a study is seriously flawed.

Your evaluation of an article should primarily focus on four domains: (1) measurement, (2) internal validity, (3) external validity, and (4) data analysis. You may encounter issues in other domains (e.g., ethical considerations), but most issues can be put into one of these four areas.

In terms of measurement (see Chapter 2), the researcher should clearly describe the instruments used in the study, as well as evidence for their reliability and validity. If the researcher does not discuss this in any detail, he or she should provide a citation for other articles that do so. You should also ask if the researcher properly addresses other measurement issues that may impact the results (e.g., sensitivity, reactivity).

As we discussed in Chapter 3, internal validity is concerned with whether we can accurately infer cause-and-effect relationships. The ability to establish internal validity is largely determined by the type of research design used. Randomized controlled experiments are the best designs for establishing internal validity. Reversal (e.g., ABA, ABAB) and multiple-baseline designs also attempt to address the issue of internal validity, although sample sizes for these designs are typically quite small. Nonexperimental designs (e.g., survey research, qualitative research) typically do not offer as strong of evidence for internal validity. For example, surveys typically generate correlational data, which can lead to spurious relationships or problems in determining the direction of cause and effect. Researchers need to be careful not to overstate conclusions about cause and effect, particularly when doing nonexperimental research. Furthermore, researchers should identify potential threats to internal validity in the discussion.

When evaluating external validity (see Chapter 4), you want to evaluate the extent to which the sample is representative of the population to which you hope to generalize the findings. Generally, this requires understanding the steps the researcher took to ensure the sample was representative of the population of interest. For example, did the researcher use probability sampling (e.g., random, systematic, strata, or multistage cluster)? Or, did the researcher use nonprobability sampling (e.g., convenience sampling), which has poorer external validity? In addition, you must consider if a low response rate threatened the representativeness of the sample even if probability sampling was used. You should also determine if the sample is adequately described (e.g., demographics). This is especially important in qualitative research, where generalizability is determined by comparing the study sample to those with whom you want to apply the findings. Researchers will ideally discuss the threats to external validity in the limitations section of the discussion.

Finally, you should attempt to evaluate if data analysis was conducted properly. For quantitative research, this will require evaluating if the proper statistical techniques were used and if the analyses were properly done (see Chapters 9–11). In terms of the latter, this means evaluating if the assumptions behind the analyses were confirmed (e.g., variables are normally distributed) and issues of missing data were properly handled. Unfortunately, many studies never make explicit if these issues were addressed. Thus, you must take on faith that the researcher was attentive to these issues when conducting the analyses. For qualitative research (see Chapter 6), the researcher should clearly describe the method used to analyze the data (e.g., constant comparative method). Qualitative researchers need to describes the steps they took to ensure the trustworthiness of the data (e.g., triangulation, saturation, peer review).

Appendix II provides a list of questions you can use to evaluate research studies. The first part of the appendix lists questions that are applicable across a wide variety of designs. The second part lists questions that are specific to various research designs (e.g., experiments, surveys, qualitative research, meta-analysis). We think you will find the appendix a quick and easy resource for helping you evaluate studies. In addition to the book appendix, some EBP sites have worksheets practitioners can use to evaluate research studies. For example, the Evidence Based Medicine Toolkit (*www.ebm.med.ualberta.ca*) from the University of Alberta includes worksheets designed to help you evaluate a variety of different studies (Buckingham, Fisher, & Saunders, 2012).

CAN INDIRECT INDICATORS
OF QUALITY BE USED?

The optimal way to evaluate the quality of a study is to carefully read the article so you can determine its strengths and weaknesses in the four domains discussed above. This provides the most direct and reliable assessment of quality. However, this takes time and effort. Therefore, this section will discuss whether it is possible to use other means of evaluating the quality of a study, along with the potential pitfalls of using these short cuts.

One possible short cut is to consider the reputation of the journal in which the study appears. The assumption here is that higher-quality journals will have higher-quality studies, and that lower-quality journals will have lower-quality studies. There is probably some truth to this assumption, but only to a certain point. The top-tier journals in a discipline are more likely to have higher-quality studies overall. One reason is that top-tier journals can be the most selective in publishing articles because they typically have a high number of submissions. In addition, they usually have the leading experts in a field evaluate submissions through a peer review process to see if the studies warrant publication. As a result, you generally have greater assurance as to the quality of a study if it is published in one of the top-tier journals. However, this is not 100% foolproof because the peer review process is not infallible, even in these journals. Conversely, the risk of encountering a study of poor quality is greater among journals that do not do a blind review process, or that have a high acceptance rate (e.g., 50% and above). A study with serious or fatal flaws is more likely to slip through the cracks and get published in these journals.

One major shortcoming to basing the quality of an article on the reputation of the journal is that it will be less reliable when considering studies that are not published in top-tier journals. Many quality studies can be found in publications outside the top-tier journals given their low acceptance rates. In addition, many quality studies are published in journals that are not top-tier because the study best fits the specific focus of a particular journal. As result, one should not automatically discount a study simply because it does not appear in a top-tier journal.

If you are going to use the journal's quality as a possible indicator of article quality (remembering the caveats noted above), then how do you evaluate the quality of the journal? There are several ways you might do this, although each has its potential limitations. Faculty can recommend journals that have a strong reputation, although this can be somewhat subjective. Acceptance rates offer a more quantitative approach for evaluating a journal's reputation. Top journals typically have lower acceptance rates, with the most selective journals having acceptance rates below 20%. You can search *Cabell's Directories* using the *Psychology and Psychiatry* directory to find the acceptance rates of journals within the field. *Cabell's Directories* also indicate whether manuscripts go through a peer review process, which is an important safeguard to ensuring the quality of the publications.

Another potential indicator of a journal's quality could be its impact, which is a measure of how widely cited or used articles are within that journal. Different ways for measuring the impact of a journal have been suggested. Perhaps the most widely used is the **impact factor** reported in the *Journal Citation Reports* published by Thomson Reuters. Impact factors in the *Journal Citation Reports* are calculated by determining the number of citations found in a particular year for all eligible articles published in the 2 preceding years by the journal, and then dividing it by the number of eligible articles. For example, if the journal published 50 eligible articles for citation in 2011 and 2012, and if these articles collectively were cited 100 times during 2013, then the 2013 impact factor would be 2.0. Self-cited articles (i.e., citations of those articles within the same journal) are not included in the number of citations. Another measure sometimes used to measure journal impact is the **h-index**. This represents the h-number of articles that have been cited at least h times by an author, a group of authors, or a journal. For example, an h-index of 15 would mean an author has least 15 articles that have been cited a minimum of 15 times or more. Other ways of calculating a journal's impact have also been suggested and studied (Bollen, Van de Sompel, Hagberg, & Chute, 2009).

There is a lively debate on what is the best way to measure the impact of a journal, which accounts for why multiple measures have been developed. Although the impact factor in the *Journal Citation Reports* is most widely recognized, it has also been criticized for a number of reasons. For example, Burke and Phillips (2012) noted that the vast majority of citations for the most widely cited articles in *Clinical Neurophysiology* and *Muscle & Nerve* were found 2 years after publication. Therefore, impact factors may not completely capture the impact of articles given that the full extent of their citations may not be known until after 2 years. Impact ratings, like the impact factor, can also be influenced by other factors such as the type of articles they publish or the field in which they are in (Bordons, Fernández, & Gómez, 2002; Vucovich, Baker, & Smith, 2008). For example, journals that print more reviews of the literature are likely to have higher impact ratings because reviews are more likely to be cited. There are also concerns that journals can manipulate impact ratings to increase the journal's prestige. As a result, one must be cautious in using impact ratings as a sole indicator of journal quality. Impact ratings will ideally be used along with other information about the journal (e.g., acceptance rates, utlilization of blind review) to evelute the quality of the journal.

An assumption behind using journal impact ratings to evaluate individual studies is that higher-quality studies will be more likely to be cited, thus resulting in higher impact ratings for a journal. There is some support for this assumption based on the medical literature. Saha, Saint, and Christakis (2003) found there was a strong correlation between the impact factor and perceived quality of general medical journals as rated by researchers and internal medicine practitioners. Similarly, a strong correlation was found between the perceived quality of clinical neurology journals and their impact ratings (Yue, Wilson, & Boller, 2007). In addition, Lokker et al. (2012) found the quality of articles within medical journals was a predictor of its later impact factor.

Despite this association, it is important to recognize that a high impact rating for a journal does not guarantee a specific study within that journal will be of high impact or high quality. The impact rating for articles within a journal can vary significantly. Most articles are infrequently cited, while a small percentage of articles can be widely cited (Vucovich et al., 2008). Furthermore, although Gludd, Sørensen, Gøtzsche, and Gluud (2005) found impact factors could be a rough indicator of quality in medical clinical trials, they still found clinical trials within high impact journals that had small samples or inadequate quality.

Ultimately, your hope is that journals with high impact ratings are the most selective in screening and publishing studies. As a result, your assurance of the quality of a study is probably greatest when reviewing articles in journals that have high impact ratings, low acceptance rates, and use multiple blind reviewers. However, as noted above, this is not an infallible indicator of quality. In addition, only a subset of articles you may want to review will be found within these top-tier or high impact journals. So, it is still important that you be able to evaluate the strength of a study directly.

Another possible short cut is to search for studies done by researchers who have established a strong reputation in the field. This may be an effective strategy if there are some well-known researchers within the area you are exploring. Stronger researchers will typically have multiple publications in an area because they are often conducting programmatic research, including some publications within the top journals. In addition, researchers who have obtained external research funding from the government (e.g., NIH, NIMH) are often very strong due to the competitive nature of obtaining this type of funding. However, many quality studies are conducted by researchers who have not established a leading reputation in the field. Therefore, relying just on the reputation of the researcher could lead you to overlook some important and good quality research.

A third possible way of evaluating the quality of a study is to read the limitations section typically included in the discussion. In our opinion, you need to be very cautious about using this approach to evaluate the quality of a study. Our observation has been that strong researchers are usually best at recognizing and stating the limitations of their research. In contrast, weaker researchers may be more likely to overlook key limitations, or they may not even address them at all. Therefore, we recommend that you not rely solely on this as a means for evaluating the potential weaknesses of a study.

If you are going to read a variety of studies to extract key themes, then perhaps relying on one or more of the indirect indicators of quality may be sufficient, particularly if you are reading literature from mostly top-tier journals. However, if you are going to use a particular study to inform an important clinical decision, then we believe you should directly evaluate the quality of the study rather than rely on the indirect methods above. This is the most reliable way to evaluate the quality of a study. We need to carefully weigh the strength of evidence provided by the research if we are going to use it to influence our clients' lives.

READING AND EVALUATING
A SYSTEMATIC REVIEW

A literature review of many studies, often referred to as a systematic review, is a summary of the best available research in a particular area of concern. Systematic reviews can be a helpful resource for busy clinicians who need good-quality information on the effectiveness and appropriateness of a particular intervention (e.g., acceptance and commitment therapy in marital therapy), but don't have time due to their heavy clinical caseload to sift through a large number of studies that may offer unclear, confusing, or contradictory results. The exponential increase of research literature in the areas of mental health and mental health services, along with the information explosion on the Internet and social media, make it almost impossible for therapists to keep up with current information and decipher the quality of evidence presented.

Similar to individual research studies, systematic reviews of the literature use rigorous, transparent methods to minimize bias in results. Systematic reviews are not the same as traditional literature reviews of convenience or journalistic reviews, which is the usual method used by students in papers written for particular courses, and are also seen in medical review articles (e.g., UpToDate). Journalistic reviews often use selectively chosen research studies or conceptual essays that have not been identified or analyzed in a systematic, unbiased way. Systematic reviews have clear, explicit objectives and methods with clearly stated inclusion criteria for studies to be selected, use systematic searching methods that reduce the risk of selective sampling of studies, and use consistent evaluation of available information. In addition, systematic reviews are explicit and transparent enough to enable someone else to reproduce the method. When available, it's ideal to use a systematic review rather than a journalistic review of the literature. However, non-systematic reviews can also be helpful as long as you are aware of the limitations.

Based on the work of Greenhalgh (2010) and O'Connor, Whitlock, and Spring (2012), we suggest you ask the following questions in your assessment of systematic reviews:

1. Can you find an important clinical question which the review addressed? A systematic review should include a precise question to be answered by the literature, which dictates what research will be included or excluded in the review.

2. Was a thorough search done of the appropriate database(s) with a particular strategy and were other potentially important sources explored? If only one database was used, it's highly likely that relevant articles were missed. Searching a database requires the use of well-thought out combinations of keywords. Even when the right keywords have been entered, it's highly unlikely that all the relevant papers will be found in one database, which is why the best systematic reviews of the literature use many databases in their search. In addition to multiple databases, researchers are often searching the references of identified papers, and the references of the references (Greenhalgh, 2010).

3. Were there explicit inclusion/exclusion criteria reported that were related to selection of the primary studies? For example, did the study include or exclude studies on children?

4. How many reviewers were involved, were the studies examined independently, and how were disagreements resolved? Is there any evidence the process was biased or inadequately implemented?

5. Was methodological quality assessed? The process for evaluating quality should be explained.

6. Is sufficient detail of the individual studies presented? The review should include a table giving information on design and results of studies (in addition to) narrative descriptions of the studies within the text.

7. Are the primary studies summarized appropriately? There should be a narrative summary of results, which may be accompanied by a quantitative summary.

8. Is there a transparent system to evaluate the quality of body of evidence? Were the authors' conclusions supported by the evidence they presented? Authors should point out strengths and weaknesses, and offer an assessment of their confidence in the conclusions.

You may find journalistic reviews that include some of the attributes of a systematic review. Therefore, the questions suggested above for systematic reviews can also be used to evaluate journalistic reviews. The more closely a journalistic review approximates a systematic review based on the criteria above, the more confident you can be in the quality of the review.

WHERE TO FIND SYSTEMATIC REVIEWS

A good place to start looking for systematic reviews is the Cochrane Database of Systematic Reviews (CDSR), which is updated regularly at *www.cochrane.org*. Also part of the Cochrane library, the Database of Abstracts of Review of Effects (DARE; *www.crd.york.ac.uk/crdweb*) is a database of systematic reviews focused primarily on the effects of health care interventions and the delivery of health services, as well as wider determinants of health, such as housing, transportation, and social support that have a potential impact on health. If you are looking for systematic reviews in the areas of education, criminal justice, international development, and social welfare, the Campbell Collaboration (C2; *www.campbellcollaboration.org*) is a good resource. To broaden your search, you can go to PsycInfo or Google Scholar and include "systematic review" along with your other keywords. An example is provided in the next section.

CASE ILLUSTRATIONS OF USING A SINGLE STUDY AND SYSTEMATIC REVIEWS

Vignette 1: Use of a Single Study

Jayden is working with Ashton and Reese in couple therapy to address ongoing conflict. Reese has been recently diagnosed with borderline personality disorder (BPD), which Jayden believes has been contributing to the conflict in the couple's marriage. Jayden remembers reading in his couple therapy course how dialectical behavior therapy (DBT) principles had been applied to couples where one individual had BPD (Fruzetti & Fantozzi, 2008). He believes this approach might be a good fit for Ashton and Reese, but wonders if there is any empirical support for this treatment.

Using PsycINFO, Jayden discovers a recent outcome study that evaluated DBT couple therapy with an Iranian sample (Kamalabadi et al., 2012). Jayden notices the study is published in the *Interdisciplinary Journal of Contemporary Research in Business*, which is obviously not a top journal within the psychotherapy field. Jayden realizes he will not be able to rely on the reputation of the journal as an indicator of quality, so he must read the article to directly evaluate its quality.

Jayden notes that one key strength is that the study used a randomized controlled trial (RCT) to evaluate the treatment. This gives him greater confidence in the internal validity of the findings. The study briefly but adequately describes the instruments used in the study, including evidence for the reliability of the instruments based on Iranian samples. The analyses seem appropriate, although no details are offered on whether the assumptions behind the analyses were tested. Jayden's most significant concerns relate to external validity. In this study, all of the individuals diagnosed with BPD are male. Jayden questions if the findings will apply if the female is diagnosed with BPD, which is more commonly the case. In addition, Jayden wonders if having an Iranian sample will impact his ability to generalize the findings to his clients. Nonetheless, the study appears to be strong enough to support trying a DBT approach with Ashton and Reese.

Vignette 2: Use of Systematic Reviews

Shannon is working with the Jansen family, who are seeking help in coping with the death of Marcus (age 11), who died 6 months earlier when he was hit by a car while riding his bicycle. Shannon has been working on bereavement issues with the family, but is particularly concerned about Ian (age 9) because he witnessed the accident. Ian has become more anxious since the accident, and reports frequent nightmares where he relives the experience of seeing Marcus die. Shannon wonders if Ian needs to be specifically treated for the trauma he witnessed above and beyond the grief work she is doing with the family. She is aware that eye movement desensitization and reprocessing (EMDR) is an approach that is sometimes used with adults to deal with trauma. However, she is uncertain how effective EMDR is, and whether it can be used effectively with children.

Shannon looks for research to answer her questions. First, Shannon searches the *Cochrane Database of Systematic Reviews* and finds a systematic review on the psychological treatment of PTSD by Bisson and Andrew (2009). In this review, the authors noted that trauma-focused cognitive-behavioral therapy and EMDR have the strongest empirical support for treating PTSD. Although this review gives Shannon more confidence that EMDR might be effective in dealing with Ian's trauma, she is still uncertain as to how effective EMDR is with children or adolescents. Therefore, Shannon tries to locate a systematic review on the use of EMDR with children. By using the keywords *systematic review, eye movement desensitization, and reprocessing,* and *children* in the PsycINFO database, she finds a systematic review on the use of EMDR with children and adolescents by Field and Cottrell (2011). The review suggests EMDR might be effective with children or adolescents, although more research in this area is clearly warranted. Shannon concludes there is sufficient evidence to suggest that making a referral for EMDR to treat Ian's trauma is worthwhile. Furthermore, in light of the empirical evidence she has read, Shannon is contemplating getting trained in EMDR so she can treat future clients with trauma using this approach.

CONCLUSION

The ability to critically evaluate the quality of a study is a valuable and necessary skill in EBP. Without the ability to appraise the quality of a study, we are unable to determine the level of confidence we should have in the research. Similarly, it is important that we are able to assess the quality of systematic reviews, which can be a valuable and time-saving way for the busy clinician to learn about research in a particular area. In the next chapter, we will discuss some of the challenges you may face as you translate research findings into clinical practice.

CHAPTER 15

Apply I

Translating Research Findings into Clinical Practice

Once you know which treatment approaches have empirical support (Step 3, "Appraise"; see Chapter 14), you are still left with the question of how to implement these approaches into your clinical work (Beutler, 2000). It is often at this stage in the process that the knowledge gained from research is combined with creativity and clinical expertise to develop appropriate treatment plans for our clients. In Step 4, we combine our clinical expertise, patient preferences, and clinical context. Clinical expertise includes what we know and what we do not know. For example, a therapist might have been trained in multisystemic therapy but know nothing about emotionally focused therapy because she did her internship at a drug abuse clinic for adolescents. After conducting a search and realizing that you know little about the research-supported treatment model, you may be motivated to learn that model.

Our clients bring us their stories, other experiences with past-therapies, and personal beliefs. A Christian client might be open to a specific therapy as long as the therapist is also a professing Christian. Another client may adamantly oppose taking psychotropic medications because a family member had a bad experience with medications many years ago. Clients might have limited insurance, finances, time, and energy. Clinics may have mandates to follow specific treatments and guidelines due to resource allocation. All of these factors have to be considered when treatment choices are made and implemented.

The utility of EBP rests on the generalizability of basic clinical science findings and the fidelity of implementation (the therapist's ability to do the specific treatment). Consequently, the transportability of RCTs has been hotly debated in the literature (e.g., Chambless & Hollon, 1998; Franklin & DeRubeis, 2006; Westen, 2006a) and is now the focus of a burgeoning area of science called *translational research*. For example, clinicians interested in translational research want to know if the tightly controlled treatment protocol of an RCT can be used in the messy world of clinical practice. In this chapter, we discuss the challenges inherent in applying research clinically, especially as it relates to using outcome research to inform treatment plans in the real world (Norcross, Beutler, & Levant, 2006). We will primarily organize this chapter around key questions you will want to ask yourself as you apply research to your clinical practice.

FACTORS THAT PREDICT THERAPY EFFECTIVENESS BESIDES THE SPECIFIC TREATMENT MODEL

Most of the evidence-based literature focuses on specific models, treatment protocols, and manualized interventions (Chambless et al., 1996). However, research has also indicated that other variables strongly influence therapy outcomes regardless of what interventions are used. In fact, the client–therapist relationship consisting of the trust and belief that the therapist cares about the individual and has the ability to help are often important factors influencing treatment outcomes (Lambert, 2013). Therapists that ignore these softer "relationship" factors, even while they strictly adhere to an EBP treatment manual, may find that their clients fail to make progress. In Chapter 18, we discuss ways therapists can assess the therapeutic alliance. Common factors such as the client's motivation to change also influence treatment outcomes (Sprenkle, 2004), and should not be ignored.

"HOW DOES MY CLIENT COMPARE TO THE SAMPLES UPON WHICH THE RESEARCH WAS CONDUCTED?"

The client that appears in your office will in all likelihood deviate in important ways from research samples (Kent & Hayward, 2007). Outcome research focuses on establishing internal validity (Chapter 3), but by doing so, the generalizability of the findings or external validity (Chapter 4) can be compromised. Even the most ecologically valid RCTs have such strict inclusion criteria that the sample participants are not representative of the general clinical population (Westen, 2006a). For instance, in the National Institute of Mental Health (NIMH) Treatment of Adolescent Depression Study (TADS; March et al., 2004) researchers examined the efficacy of fluoexetine (Prozac), cognitive-behavior therapy, and the combination of the two, in comparison to a placebo control condition. Participants in this study were excluded if they endorsed suicidality, substance abuse, problematic school attendance, bipolar diagnosis, psychiatric hospitalizations, and residence with someone other than a primary caretaker. Furthermore, participants had to meet the diagnostic criteria for major depressive disorder over the course of multiple screenings. Interestingly, the TADS had far less restrictive criteria than the average controlled study of adolescent depression. In fact, the average RCT excludes 30–70% of patients screened for inclusion (Westen, Novotny, & Thomas-Brenner, 2004). In clinical practice, variation in presentation and comorbidity is the rule rather than the exception, making the findings of some studies far less generalizable than one might originally assume.

For all the reasons presented above and more, RCTs alone should never determine the treatment plan. Rather, clinical expertise is always required to successfully implement EBPs. The clinician determines the applicability of research to a particular case after thorough assessment and communication with the client about preferences and goals.

Family therapists also face a unique challenge. In clinical trials of couple or family treatments, researchers require specific family members to participate in order to be included in the study. Often, clinicians do not have the ability to require specific family members to participate. The fidelity of the intervention may then be compromised. Also, which family members actually show up each week might vary. In addition, the family may not agree on a treatment plan and may not even agree on who should come to therapy.

Thus, in many ways, your clients may differ from the research samples. But we do not recommend that you abandon the evidence-based treatments. Clinical work can be messy and ambiguous at times. We hope that you will make it your goal to approximate the treatment protocol as closely as possible, while maintaining clinical flexibility in addressing situational challenges.

"HOW WILL I KNOW IF IT WORKS
IN THE REAL WORLD?"

A distinction is often made between research conducted in clinical settings and research conducted in laboratories. Experimental studies that are done in real-world clinical settings are called **effectiveness studies** whereas experimental studies that are more carefully controlled, such as a RCT, are called **efficacy studies** (see Chapter 3). Efficacy studies are prioritized above effectiveness studies when determining EBP status because they are best able to demonstrate that a treatment alone caused change in outcome. However, efficacy studies are often so rigidly controlled that they often do represent the complexities of mental health treatment in the real world. Effectiveness studies, on the other hand, have an advantage when it comes to the applicability of research because they come much closer to simulating what happens in the real world.

Effectiveness studies conducted in the later phases of the research process are usually the most beneficial for practicing clinicians. Research often starts with small case studies that incorporate client feedback and response. Once a treatment shows possibility, then larger open studies are conducted and researchers may develop specific "manualized" treatment protocols. Eventually, RCTs are conducted to demonstrate effectiveness compared to control conditions and treatment alternatives. Once efficacy has been demonstrated and replicated, researchers shift their focus to (a) examining the specific ingredients for success, (b) examining individual differences, and (c) examining moderators, such as age, gender, socioeconomic status, clinical setting, and comorbid conditions.

Thus, the ability to apply EBP treatments in everyday clinical settings has become an important empirical question examined by researchers (e.g., Tashiro & Mortensen, 2006; Wade, Treat, & Stuart, 1998; Weersing & Weisz, 2002). **Translational research** examines what happens when "research findings are moved from the researcher's bench to the patient's bedside and community" (Rubio et al., 2010, p. 4). Research in this area has only just begun, but will become especially important for therapists practicing EBP. To date, effectiveness studies of treatments for anxiety disorders and depression are encouraging; similar outcomes have been reported across clinical trials, outpatient clinics, and private practice (e.g., Franklin & DeRubeis, 2006). However, as cogently argued by Westen (2006b), the types of manualized treatments shown to be effective in efficacy studies assume that patients can be treated as if they have a single disorder or in an additive fashion, addressing multiple disorders in a step-by-step manner. In addition, other factors that influence clients, such as divorce, poverty, or bullying, might never be noted. As a therapist and an observer, you might believe that your depressed teenage client will not become less depressed until his parents stop fighting and the school bully leaves him alone regardless of the efficacy of the evidence-based treatment you are using. You are probably correct! You can still deliver the evidence-based treatment but you will have to simultaneously try to help him solve his contextual struggles.

A focus on systems rather than individual diagnoses would suggest that the context of depressed clients' lives (e.g., childhood trauma, poverty, difficult interpersonal relationships) varies and is as important a focus of treatment as the symptoms themselves. Also, multiple family members may bring multiple confounding influences to the therapy room. The father may be unemployed, the mother may have a chronic illness, and the identified patient may not want to be in therapy at all.

As systems-oriented therapists, family therapists might find themselves asking, "For whom is the research applicable and what aspects of the research should be transported?" Problems of transportability are often problems related to external validity. Another important issue is what should be transported? Should the treatment manual shown to be effective in controlled research or general principles and theory-driven techniques be applied? The answer to this question will likely depend on the problem and the treatment itself. For instance, exposure-based treatments are more amenable to standardization than emotionally focused therapy. Whether or not you decide to use a manualized treatment approach or focus on general principles, strong clinical judgment will still be important (Rosen & Davison, 2003).

"HOW DO I LEARN ABOUT AN APPROACH THAT HAS SUPPORT?"

Once you have identified an evidence-based approach you want to use, you may still be left with the issue of trying to find out enough information about it so you can actually implement it. There may be a variety of ways in which you can learn about an evidence-based treatment approach. Many of the treatments that have been tested through research have manuals that outline the treatment approach. These manuals were developed to make sure that the therapists delivered the treatment as intended. Some researchers may be willing to send you the manual upon request. In some cases, the manuals may be available on the Internet at no cost, particularly if the treatment was evaluated using federal funding (e.g., NIMH grants). Therefore, you should search the Internet to see if you can locate a treatment manual for the approach.

For some of the more popular evidence-based models, the developers may have written books that describe the treatment approach. For example, several of the evidence-based models for couple therapy (see Chapter 16) have books written for clinicians (see Appendix III). Some have even written books intended for clients based on their model. In addition, some of the models may offer specialized training through workshops that may eventually lead to being certified in that approach (e.g., Gottman Method Couple Approach, emotionally focused therapy).

"CAN I ADAPT A TREATMENT FOR MY PARTICULAR CLIENT OR CLINICAL STYLE?"

Discussions with clients about treatment options overlap with the legal principle of informed consent. Informed consent is an important issue for therapists using evidence-based treatments. In essence, informed consent gives your clients the right to know what their diagnoses are and what treatment options exist to help them. The elements of informed consent generally include (Edwards, 2008):

- A description of a treatment option.
- Other alternatives to the treatment option.
- Relevant risks, benefits, and uncertainties related to each alternative.
- Assessment of the clients' understanding.
- Consent (or not) of the treatment by the client.

Chapter 17 discusses in more detail how to talk to clients about an evidence-based approach and provides more information about informed consent.

Clients will vary on how much information they already know or need to know about evidence-based treatments. For example, some clients might want to know more about the basic research behind your treatment recommendations. You can help them find that information. For example, we know colleagues who share research articles related to a specific diagnosis or treatment with their clients who have that problem. This usually occurs when the client and therapist are a "detective team"—searching for options for some unusual problems. In addition, clients who are interested in original research are often educated, curious, and are used to doing "research" on any new problem they confront. A benefit of looking at the original research with your clients is that the shared search simultaneously builds the therapeutic relationship and convinces the client they are getting the best care possible.

Other clients may have few questions about your treatment recommendations or not even know what questions to ask. They trust your expertise. Even with these clients, it can be useful to explain that the choices you are making about their care are based on the research literature. One of our colleagues summarizes some of his key clinical questions at the end of the first session and seeks confirmation from the client that he has identified the client's key concerns. At times, he tells the client that he will research his concerns and report his results at the next session.

At the other end of the spectrum, some clients will be proactive in learning about treatment approaches. In fact, clients increasingly search the web for information about their problems and may come for therapy seeking a specific treatment. We know of many situations where clients ask if the therapist knows a particular therapy model because they have decided that is the best model for their particular problems—even before they enter your office door. Since the client's positive attitude about the treatment (belief that it will work) enhances the probability that it will work, you will want to listen carefully to your client's preferences and beliefs. If two treatments are equally effective, you should pick the treatment that your client requests.

Therapists often adapt treatments to fit the complex, real-world clinical problems that come through their doors. Modifying treatment for a particular client or clinical style is easier if the therapist focuses on general principles and techniques rather than a specific manualized protocol. Developers of manualized treatment approaches try to protect the fidelity of implementation by requiring training and supervision before a therapist can state that they are using that model in practice (e.g., multisystemic therapy). Therefore, for ethical and legal reasons, it is important to know if the specific approach you want to implement requires special training or certification. In addition, sometimes therapists seek certification to gain formal recognition for their expertise in a specific model. For example, the Gottman Institute publishes the names of therapists who have received specific training in marital therapy skills based on John Gottman's research (*www.gottmanreferralnetwork.com*).

For widely accessible treatments, it is unclear how much modification can occur while still maintaining treatment fidelity. With modification, it is sometimes unclear whether the key ingredients for successful treatment are implemented. Furthermore, if the treatment is not effective with a particular client, it may be unclear if the treatment did not work for this particular type of client or whether the therapist did not effectively implement the treatment. Therapists have varying levels of training for specific models. For example, many family therapists could identify a few models they feel highly competent using. But they can also identify models they use less frequently and feel less skilled applying.

"HOW SHOULD I COMBINE EVIDENCE-BASED TREATMENTS ON MULTIPLE PROBLEMS IN ONE CLIENT OR MULTIPLE CLIENTS IN A FAMILY?"

In general, research protocols require that variables are clearly defined and specific. Interventions, outcomes, and contextual variables are narrowly defined, which often leads to a reductionistic view of a specific problem or diagnosis. As mentioned earlier, subjects whose problems might be too complex are often excluded from research focused on a specific clinical problem. In contrast, your clients enter your office with multiple concerns; and in families, each member might have a different view of the problem and the solution. Before you search for the evidence, you have to reach some consensus on the problem definition. Often, the easiest problem definition for an evidence-based search will be a DSM diagnosis. For example, Mr. Jones, Mrs. Jones, and Tommy all agree that he has ADHD because the school psychologist told them he did. They come to therapy seeking treatment for Tommy so he can make better grades. At first, this might seem like a straightforward case that will be a good match for evidence-based treatment. You can do a search on evidence-based treatments for ADHD and find many helpful suggestions. But perhaps the Jones family's needs might be more complex. Mr. Jones is unemployed and you suspect he has ADHD as well. The Jones family may lose their home because they cannot make their payments and Tommy would have to change school districts if they did. Also, Mrs.

Jones's brother was killed in a tragic accident 6 months earlier and she has been unable to sleep or work much since his death.

Evidence-based treatment does not always capture the complex challenges clients face. Thus, as the family's therapist, you have to create a comprehensive treatment plan with as much guidance from the EBP literature as possible. Student therapists often report the feedback they get on a specific case varies depending on the number of supervisors and colleagues they seek feedback from and the number of problems they identify.

Talking to multiple supervisors can be confusing initially. But, over time, each therapist learns to draw from multiple sources to create the best treatment plan possible for his clients. In like manner, you might end up doing several searches on several topics to create the Jones's treatment plan. Ultimately, you and the Joneses will decide the treatment priorities and possibilities.

In the case of the Jones family, here are some possible topics you could explore using the evidence-based literature:

- Tommy—treatment for ADHD, school support for ADHD students.
- Mrs. Jones—complicated grief, depression.
- Mr. Jones—treatment of adult ADHD.
- Family—effects of stress pile up on family functioning including unemployment, financial stress, and moving.

When combining different evidence-based treatments into a treatment plan, it may be helpful to think through how the different treatments may relate to one another. In some cases, you may discover that the same evidence-based treatment can be used for more than one problem. For example, cognitive-behavioral therapy could be used for treating both depression and anxiety. However, in most cases you will likely need to use two or more evidence-based treatments to treat multiple problems. In some instances, the effects of one treatment will not impact the effects of the other treatment. In other cases, however, you need to be aware that the treatments may interact (e.g., like how medications sometimes do). If this happens, ideally the treatments will complement one another and yield a synergistic effect. Yet, it is also possible that there could be a negative interaction between two evidence-based treatments. For example, if you are working with a couple that is having problems in their marriage, you may discover the husband is depressed and has low sexual desire. For the marital difficulties, you might decide to use an evidence-based approach like emotionally focused therapy or integrative behavioral couple therapy (see Chapter 16). To treat the depressive symptoms, you might consider an antidepressant or cognitive-behavioral therapy. In this particular case, however, you may avoid recommending an antidepressant because you recognize that a common side effect of antidepressants is reduced sexual desire. Therefore, you might decide to first try an evidence-based course of couple treatment to see if improving the relationship alleviates the symptoms of depression and sexual desire or perhaps suggest cognitive-behavioral therapy as an adjunct for treating the depressive symptoms.

CONCLUSION

This chapter discusses translating research into clinical practice. In essence, you are the translator. You can use information about therapeutic process and translational science to help you translate the research findings. For example, regardless of the evidence-based treatment choice, you want to always remember the critical importance of a strong therapeutic relationship. Also, you want to make sure you use language that your client understands and you share the decision making about the treatment(s) with your client. If you pay attention to the therapeutic relationship while practicing evidence-based treatments, you can be sure that your client is receiving excellent care.

CHAPTER 16

Apply II

Utilizing Couple and Family
Therapy Research in Clinical Practice

April recently finished her first semester of training at a family therapy masters program. April states that her favorite class was focused on family therapy theories, which covered a variety of approaches. She could clearly see how she would use these theories in her future clinical work. Her least favorite course, however, was Research Methods. She shares that she finds research a little boring, and is also a little intimidated by reading research studies. April candidly admits that she has a hard time seeing herself searching for and reading a lot of research articles in the future.

Ambivalence about the role of science is not unique to family therapists. Baker, McFall, and Shoham (2008) criticized clinical psychologists for valuing personal experience over science and not using interventions that carry strong evidence of efficacy. They claim that the typical clinical psychologist often lacks information on whether a specific treatment is better than placebo and views research as having little relevance to their clinical decision making (Lucock, Hall, & Noble, 2006; Nunez, Poole, & Memon, 2003). The same criticisms could be directed at mental health professionals in a variety of disciplines, including family therapy (Dattilio et al., 2014).

In an effort to learn more about the strategies therapists actually use in therapy, Garland et al. (2010) studied 1,215 video-recorded sessions of child-focused therapy led by 100 clinicians from a variety of mental health professions, including licensed systems-oriented marital and family therapists. They learned that real-world therapists use a wide variety of treatment strategies, but with less depth and low levels of intensity. They use several low-intensity elements of evidence-based practice frequently, such as psychoeducation and goal setting, and other elements less frequently, such as homework and role playing. The bad news from this study is that therapists don't use some evidence-based strategies at all or with enough intensity (and may not know whether the strategies they're using are evidence based or not). The good news from this study is that therapists are using some evidence-based strategies.

Attempts to bridge research and the practice of marriage and family therapy have historically generated controversy and passionate debate. As self-identified mavericks of the mental health establishment, family therapists have questioned the usefulness of research that focuses on individual therapy for treating mental health disorders, which ignores the complexity of interacting relational systems (e.g., couple/marital, parent–child, intergenerational, and larger system relationships) and families coping with multiple problems. Oftentimes, the populations studied in research don't accurately reflect the complexity of multi-problem families seen by family therapists and runs counter to the systems-based clinical training that is characteristic of most family therapy training programs. Sexton et al. (2011) aptly summarize the challenge:

> The clinical work of couple and family therapy is based on a unique set of relationally based principles and practices that require a different system of evaluation (e.g., change criteria, variability of methodological approaches, types of analyses) than does individual therapy. For example, the most common problems for which people seek couple and family therapy (such as "family" problems involving high levels of conflict but without a designated or diagnosed "patient" or extramarital affairs) have never been examined to determine efficacious or effective treatments. (p. 379)

As a result, family therapists in the trenches have sometimes asked, "What does the research have to do with me and my work with couples and families?" Thus, April, the student described at the beginning of the chapter, may not be alone in expressing reservations about the relevance of research to clinical work.

Is April (and others like her), a lost cause in terms of developing her into an evidence-based practitioner? We argue that the answer is no.

One way April can incorporate evidence-based practice into her clinical work is to learn theories or treatment models that have empirical support. If she invests time and energy in learning some of these models, which she sees as having clinical relevance, then she can become a consumer of research.

April can use a variety of sources to identify evidence-based treatments that she may want to learn. For example, Division 12 of the American Psychological Association has created a website (*www.div12. org/PsychologicalTreatments*) that lists various evidenced-based treatments for treating many adult psychological disorders. For each disorder, a brief description of the disorder is provided, along with various psychological treatments that have been evaluated. The level of research support for each treatment (e.g., strong support, modest support) is noted. A brief description of the treatment is also available. The large majority of treatments described on this site are individually oriented treatments, which is consistent with a focus on individual psychopathology.

Division 53 of the American Psychological Association has a website (*www.effectivechildtherapy.com*) that focuses specifically on child and adolescent disorders. Like the other site, possible evidence-based treatments for each disorder are listed, along with the level of evidence for each. Treatments are classified as being well-established, probably efficacious, possibly efficacious, or experimental, based on the level of empirical support. The site also provides a brief description for many of the treatments, which include individual, group, and family-based treatments.

The American Psychiatric Association also has a website (*www. psych.org/practice/clinical-practice-guidelines*) that offers practice guidelines for treating various psychiatric illnesses for adults. For treating children and adolescent disorders, one can consult the American Academy of Child and Adolescent Psychiatry's website (*www.aacap.org/AACAP/ Resources_for_Primary_Care/Practice_Parameters_and_Resource_Centers/ Practice_Parameters.aspx*). Their practice guidelines also include recommendations for screening or assessing children and adolescents for these disorders. As one might expect, practice guidelines for these two sites place a heavy emphasis on using medications for treating psychiatric disorders.

Although the above are valuable resources, they are incomplete in addressing the needs of family therapists. Family therapists often treat other issues besides just psychological disorders. For example, family therapists often work with couples in distress, and therefore need guidance on treating couples from an evidence-based perspective. Even when they do work with psychological disorders, family therapists are often interested in treating them from a relational perspective. Therefore, this chapter will discuss evidence-based treatments that are couple and family based so that family therapists can effectively treat common issues they may encounter in clinical practice. However, before describing these treatments, we will first explore why learning couple- and family-based treatments is so important.

WHY FAMILY- AND COUPLE-BASED TREATMENTS MATTER

Regardless of theoretical orientation, family therapists share the core belief that relationships are important in overall health and need attention in the therapy room. The literature is replete with research documenting the correlation between relationship quality, health, and mental health. In his book *Social Intelligence*, Daniel Goleman (2007) underscores this point when he states that "relationships cut two ways: they can buffer us from illness or intensify the ravages of aging and disease" (p. 224). Goleman describes many studies that show the harmful effects of troubled relationships and the biological benefits that emerge from nurturing relationships. Poor relationships are as dangerous to our health as smoking, high blood pressure, obesity, and physical inactivity (Kiecolt-Glaser, Glaser, & Malarkey, 1999).

In his seminal work on social relationships and health, Sheldon Cohen from the University of Pittsburgh has demonstrated how environmental variables, such as social support (e.g., emotional support) and social integration (e.g., participation in a broad range of social activities or relationships) are beneficial to health (Cohen, 2004). For individuals with high stress levels, social connections provide psychological and material resources for coping with that stress. When we perceive that others will provide appropriate aid under stressful conditions, our perceived ability to cope with life's demands is enhanced, lowering the stress that these demands impose and decreasing the risk for physical and psychiatric disorders. A good example is Cohen's research on susceptibility to the common cold: When individuals participate in more types of social relationships (e.g., friends, family, work, community), they show greater resistance to upper respiratory illness (Cohen, Doyle, Skoner, Rabin, & Gwaltney, 1997).

For many adults, the most important social relationship they have is with an intimate partner. Therefore, the couple relationship is also arguably the most influential relationship on physical and mental health in adults (Keitner, Heru, & Glick, 2010). Research on marriage has been quite consistent and mirrors Cohen's findings on the importance of social relationships: As the central relationship for most adults, marriage can be a buffer for a range of emotional and physical illnesses, including mood disorders, anxiety disorders, substance use disorders, cancer, dementia, and heart attacks (Whisman & Ubelacker, 2006). Heightened strain in marriage erodes this buffer, reduces needed support, and has the potential to add repeated, chronic social stress that jeopardizes individual and relational well-being, including emotional and physical distress.

Recovery from cardiac illness provides a helpful example: Spouses can provide much needed support to improve functioning, but their own caregiving stress, including fears of their spouse dying, can diminish one's ability to be supportive. When spouses are more distressed, they are more hypervigilant of their spouse's health and controlling of their spouse's behavior (So & LaGuardia, 2011). Interventions that focus on the individual recovering from illness *and* the spouse and relationship are critical in optimizing treatment.

Beyond its impact on physical health, the literature provides ample evidence demonstrating a link between couple relationships and individual emotional well-being (Beach & Whisman, 2012). Proulx, Helms, & Buehler (2007) conducted a meta-analysis of 93 studies and found that marital quality is positively related to personal well-being over time. This finding is consistent with an earlier meta-analysis showing a relationship between marital satisfaction and depression (Whisman, 2001).

Family therapists have always believed that relationships are central to emotional and physical well-being and are central to our work as therapists. The research described above gives empirical support for that belief. Thus, as family therapists, we should be well-versed in evidence-based treatments for treating relationships.

UTILIZING EVIDENCE-BASED TREATMENTS IN FAMILY THERAPY

Since 1995, the *Journal of Marital and Family Therapy* has published three research reviews of family-based interventions for specific family problems, including conduct disorder and delinquency in adolescents, drug abuse, child and adolescent disorders, alcoholism, couples distress, intimate partner violence, affective disorders, and physical health problems. In the 2003 review, a meta-analysis reported that family therapy is clearly efficacious in comparison to no treatment and at least as efficacious as other forms of therapy, such as individual therapy (Shadish & Baldwin, 2003). The study also concluded that there's not much difference in efficacy among the many approaches to family therapy. Although this information is validating and comforting to family therapists and enables them to communicate the general effectiveness of what they do, it doesn't provide a specific guide to family therapists in their daily practice (Carr, 2012). The contemporary family therapist interested in the integration of science in her practice needs information on the most effective family therapy models and interventions.

Below, we briefly summarize the most effective family therapy models and interventions and then provide a summary of the common threads of these approaches. These approaches are considered the gold standard of family therapy because of the research methodology used to study their effectiveness (Sprenkle, 2012): randomized controlled trials (RCTs). We focus on evidence-based treatment models in this chapter because clinicians often are most interested in knowing what treatments are effective based on research. However, we do not mean to imply that this is the only valid way to use research to inform our clinical work. Furthermore, there is a great deal of research outside the family therapy field that can be helpful to our work. We agree with Lebow (2006), who states that research focused on a problem or family type can have as much clinical relevance as research on family therapy. Unfortunately, an exhaustive summary of all the family research relevant to family therapists is beyond the scope of this book. Our hope is that this general overview will familiarize you with important evidence-based approaches in the family therapy field and encourage you to explore the models in more detail for use in your practice. You will find a list of books in Appendix III that you can reference if you are interested in learning more about the approaches described hereafter.

Children and Adolescents as the Presenting Problem

Of all the family therapy approaches studied to date, the most impressive results have emerged from integrative models that address serious conduct and drug-related problems in adolescence: functional family therapy, brief strategic family therapy, multisystemic therapy, and multidimensional family therapy. We will briefly describe each approach, summarize their commonalities, and then discuss additional evidence-based approaches to treating other child-focused problems.

Functional family therapy (FFT) has been shown to be effective for conduct disorder and adolescent delinquency (Henggeler & Sheidow, 2012). FFT is a highly intensive, team approach that takes place in both office and home settings over a 4- to 6-month period. FFT therapists begin with a strong focus on engaging families, and increasing their motivation to participate in the therapy process and undertake necessary behavior changes. FFT targets negative, oftentimes chaotic, family interactions and moves toward replacing them with more effective patterns of behavior. Interventions come from a variety of family therapy models and include anything that helps create effective patterns of behavior, such as reframing, implementing problem-solving skills, and strengthening communication.

Brief strategic family therapy (BSFT) has been shown to be effective for conduct disorder and adolescent delinquency and adolescent drug abuse (Henggeler & Sheidow, 2012; Rowe, 2012). Based on structural and strategic models of family therapy, BSFT is based on a belief that maladaptive family interactions play a key role in contributing to the development of behavior problems and are a primary target for intervention in therapy. Like FFT, BSFT strives to improve children's behavioral problems by targeting maladaptive family interactions that may be exacerbating a child's symptoms. Like structural family therapy, an emphasis is placed on joining, diagnosing problematic interactions, highlighting family strengths, and restructuring the family system. A common intervention, which also is consistent with structural therapy, is restructuring family interaction in session via coaching.

Multisystemic therapy (MST) has been shown to be effective for conduct disorder and adolescent delinquency, drug abuse, and physical health problems (Henggeler & Sheidow, 2012; Rowe, 2012; Shields, Finley, Chawla, & Meadors, 2012). MST gets its name from a belief that children are nested in multiple systems, both within the family and outside the family (e.g., peer, neighborhood, school), and is designed to make positive changes in these nested systems. Eschewing traditional models of psychotherapy that include one therapist, an office, and a 50-minute session, MST is conducted by a team of therapists that carry a caseload of four to six families that provide intensive treatment over the course of 3–5 months in settings convenient for the family, such as their home or school. MST is similar to FFT in its highly engaged approach and emphasis on altering family interaction, but has an expanded interest on relationships and activities outside of the family. Although treatment is tailored to each family, MST usually focuses on three problem areas: (1) ineffective parenting practices; (2) contact with deviant peers; and (3) poor academic performance. Ecologically based family therapy (Slesnick & Prestopnick, 2005), which is similar to MST, has also been shown to be effective with substance abusing adolescents.

Multidimensional family therapy (MDFT) has been shown to be effective for adolescent drug abuse (Rowe, 2012). Like the models described above, MDFT therapists initially work toward building a strong alliance with the family. MDFT shares many features with MST, particularly the emphasis on relationships both within the family and multiple systems that are connected to the family. Assessment and treatment strategies target four dimensions: the child, the parent(s), including the self of the parent, the family, and extrafamilial or community systems, including connections with peers, schools, and potentially, the legal system. In the adolescent dimension, adolescents are helped to develop problem-solving skills and better regulate emotions; improve social competence; and establish alternatives to substance use and delinquency. In the parent dimension, the focus is on improving parenting practices and addressing potential personal issues, such as drug abuse. The family dimension emphasizes decreasing family conflict, deepening emotional attachments, and improving family communication and problem-solving skills. In the extrafamilial domain, MDFT attempts to increase competency in interactions with the community.

Because most clinicians can't use some of the treatments described above in their pure form, it's fair to ask the question "What skills can be gleaned from these empirically supported treatments?" All four models share much in common. First, they are integrative. By integrative, we don't mean eclectic where they use one model in Session 1 and another model in Session 2 or 3. Rather, they integrate theory in their attentiveness to multiple systems: the individual, the couple/marital, family, and community. They borrow from multiple systemic and nonsystemic couple and family therapy models, including structural family therapy, strategic family therapy, and cognitive-behavioral therapy. Second, they emphasize joining skills, a therapeutic alliance, and active engagement of the therapist. Therapists don't take a passive approach; they are simultaneously providing support, leadership, and direction to mobilize the family toward desired changes. Third, they focus on structural change and the disruption of dysfunctional patterns, both within and outside the family, during and outside the sessions. Fourth, they emphasize the importance of looking at peers and developing a prosocial group of friends. Finally, they are adaptable; the models are tailored to what families need.

In addition to the models described above, additional family-based interventions have been shown to be effective for other child-related problems. Parent management training (PMT) and Parent-Child Interaction Therapy (PCIT) have both been shown to be effective in addressing common problems in children, including oppositional defiant disorder, attention deficit hyperactivity disorder, and conduct disorder. PCIT engages parents in play therapy activities with their children with the goal of enhancing the parent–child relationship, followed by parents leading the child's activity while providing consistent consequences for child cooperation or disobedience (Brinkmeyer & Eyberg, 2003; Chase & Eyberg, 2008). PMT also targets the parent–child relationship by helping parents develop skills to change their child's behavior at home (Kazdin, 2005). Treatment focuses on educating parents about social learning principles and techniques (e.g., rewarding positive behavior) and coaching parents in implementing the procedures at home. The goals of both PCIT and PMT are to diminish the presence of negative, maladaptive behaviors and reward adaptive behaviors with positive attention.

Finally, the Maudsley approach has been shown to be effective for anorexia nervosa. Maudsley is a family-based approach strongly influenced by structural family therapy that engages parents in the treatment of adolescents with eating disorders. In addition to psychoeducation about the harmful effects of starvation, a few of the key family-oriented features include (1) defining the family as a resource for helping their child rather than as a cause of the illness, (2) helping the parents take control of re-nutrition without criticism, and (3) helping the parents strengthen boundaries around their relationship (Eisler, Dare, Hodes, Russell, Dodge, & le Grange, 2000). Eisler, Simic, Russell, and Dare (2007) conducted an RCT comparing two forms of family therapy: conjoint family therapy (parents and child seen together) and separated family therapy (parents and child seen separately). They found that there was little difference in effectiveness of the treatments; both forms of family therapy resulted in more than 75% of subjects having no eating disorder symptoms. The authors did note that patients in families with high maternal criticism did less well in conjoint family therapy than separated family therapy.

PMT, PCIT, and the Maudsley model reinforce another key skill for therapists working with child-focused problems: strengthening the family hierarchy and supporting appropriate parental authority in the management of their children. In our work with family therapy students, we notice that parents are frequently on the outside of treatment looking in, as student therapists focus solely on the emotional and behavioral issues of the child. By ignoring the parents, they miss the opportunity to empower parents to take charge of their child's challenges.

Family-Based Treatments for Mental Disorders in Adulthood

Recovery from psychiatric illness is slower when family dysfunction is present. Patients with major depression, for example, have a slower rate of recovery when they live in families with significant family dysfunction. Healthy family functioning is one of the five factors associated with a good outcome in major depression (Keitner, Ryan, Miller, & Norman, 1992).

Family psychoeducation (FPE) has been shown to be effective in the treatment of severe mental illness. Led by mental health professionals, FPE is a collection of diagnostic-specific (e.g., schizophrenia, bipolar disorder) programs aimed at providing content about the illness, medication management, and treatment planning to family members as they cope with their family member's symptoms and the effects of illness on the family (Lucksted, McFarlane, Downing, Dixon, & Adams, 2012). These programs assume that (1) the actions of family members impact the person coping with illness and his treatment, and (2) family members need information and support in caring for a family member with severe mental illness (Sprenkle, 2012). Many studies from around the world have shown that FPE is effective in reducing relapse and re-hospitalization rates for individuals coping with severe mental illness, especially schizophrenia (Lucksted et al., 2012).

Behavioral couple therapy (BCT) has been shown to be effective for adult drug abuse and alcoholism (O'Farrell & Clements, 2012; Rowe, 2012). BCT works with partners conjointly with the goal of strengthening spousal support to increase the potential for sobriety, improve couple communication, and enhance enjoyable activities that don't involve substances (Rowe, 2012). The research has been quite clear that BCT is more effective than individual treatment at increasing abstinence and improving marital and family functioning (O'Farrell, 1993).

The clinical culture of most treatment programs for severe mental illness and substance abuse tends to focus on the individual patient, leaving family therapists with the dilemma of how to advocate for a systems or relational approach to treatment. The research above underscores the value of supportive family relationships in treatment. Therapists are more effective when they engage family members in treatment for drug and alcohol abuse and severe mental illness. Engaging families doesn't mean blaming them for problem behavior. Rather, engaging families allows the therapist to address relational stress that exacerbates problems. More importantly, therapists can access a family's skills and resources to help the patient in need.

Couples as the Presenting Problem

Couple therapy is obviously indicated when a couple presents specifically with marital or relationship distress. However, as discussed earlier in the chapter, couple therapy may also be a helpful approach when individuals present with physical and mental health issues. Here we will review various approaches for couple therapy that have some evidence for their effectiveness. Therapists working with couples will ideally become familiar with one or more of the following models.

Although couple and marital research has provided rich data about stress-generating processes for decades, the work of John Gottman revolutionized the way clinicians understand and treat marital relationships (Gottman, 1993). Theory-informed speculation gave way to elegant data and engaging nomenclature to explain couple distress. An exhaustive review of Gottman's research is beyond the scope of this book, but here are a few highlights from his research that every couple therapist should know:

- Conflict is a normal part of couple relationships. The focus should be on management, not extinction.
- Negative interaction that includes criticism, stonewalling, defensiveness, or contempt (four horsemen of the apocalypse) is especially problematic.
- For every one negative interaction, couples should have five positive interactions.
- Couples can benefit from down-regulating negative affect and up-regulating positive affect.
- Repairing injuries in relationships is a critical ingredient of successful couples (e.g., I'm sorry).
- Marriage benefits when a man accepts influence from his spouse.
- Intimacy, or bids for connection, can take place in ordinary moments (e.g., shared humor).

Gottman has taken these research findings and incorporated them into the Gottman Method Couple Therapy. The goals of this approach are to (1) downregulate negative affect during conflict, (2) increase positive affect during conflict, (3) build positive affect and connection outside of conflict, (4) bridge different styles for managing emotions (meta-emotion mismatches), and (5) create and nurture a shared meaning system (Gottman & Gottman, 2008). Gottman has written multiple books on his approach, including several self-help books for couples.

Integrative behavioral couple therapy (IBCT) is a newer generation of behavioral couple therapy (BCT), and has been shown to be effective for couple distress (Lebow, Chambers, Christensen, & Johnson, 2012). Although several studies have demonstrated that BCT can reduce couple distress, research also found that only about half of couples improved with BCT, and that only a third of those that improved moved into the nondistressed range (Dimidjian, Martell, & Christensen, 2008). Therefore, IBCT was developed by Neil Jacobson and Andrew Christensen in an attempt to build on the effectiveness of traditional BCT. Like its predecessor, IBCT teaches couples communication and conflict resolutions skills to reduce conflict, and encourages couples to increase caring or positive behaviors. However, IBCT also incorporates the idea of acceptance into its work with couples. IBCT tries to help couples build connection through acceptance (or at least tolerance) of their differences, rather than become polarized and trapped in conflict around them.

Emotionally focused therapy (EFT) has been shown to be effective for couple distress (Johnson, Hunsley, Greenberg, & Schindler, 1999; Lebow et al., 2012). According to EFT, due to problems in attachment, couples will (1) hide their primary emotions (e.g., fear, hurt, need for attachment) and (2) exhibit "secondary reactive emotions" (e.g., anger, defensiveness) leading to negative interaction (e.g., demand–withdraw). EFT therapists use unconditional positive regard and work with one partner at a time in the presence of the other to access primary emotions, reprocess the emotional experience of partners, and restructure interaction patterns. The experience of primary affect serves as a means for couples to *reframe* their relationship. This enables them to alter their negative interaction sequence and develop new ways of solving their problems (Johnson, 2004). Recently, EFT has expanded its focus to apply these principles in work with families, particularly parent–adolescent conflict (Johnson, 2004).

In addition to the models described above, therapists may also be interested in other approaches that have some evidence to support their effectiveness. Like IBCT described above, cognitive-behavioral couple therapy (CBCT) is a newer generation of BCT that integrates a cognitive component into the approach (Epstein & Baucom, 2002). Research suggests that CBCT has comparable effectiveness to BCT (Baucom, Epstein, LaTaillade, & Kirby, 2008). Insight-oriented couple therapy (IOCT) is another approach that has some empirical support, and is designed to help couples understand how past relationships influence their current maladaptive patterns. In one study, couples treated with IOCT were significantly less likely to have divorced 4 years after treatment compared to couples treated with BCT (Snyder, Wills, & Grady-Fletcher, 1991). Both CBCT and IOCT are the basis for an integrative treatment for addressing infidelity (Gordon, Baucom, Snyder, & Dixon, 2008). Based on a replicated case-study design, there is some promising evidence for the effectiveness of this approach for treating affairs (Gordon, Baucom, & Snyder, 2004).

REMEMBER CLIENT CONTEXT WHEN APPLYING EVIDENCE-BASED TREATMENTS

In Chapter 15, we discussed the need to tailor evidence-based treatments to the clients. A prime example of this is working with couples in stepfamilies. Although the evidence-based treatments described above are well-suited for working with couples in stepfamilies, they do not necessarily attend to all the unique needs that couples in stepfamilies may have. Stepfamilies possess unique characteristics that distinguish them from first-marriage families, including children coping with losses and loyalty binds and parenting tasks that can polarize adults (Papernow, 2008). Role ambiguity and efforts to merge multiple family cultures are complicating factors in decisions about parenting responsibilities.

Whitton, Nicholson, and Markman (2008) reviewed treatment interventions for couples in stepfamilies. A large percentage (85%) of the studies were prevention programs aimed at preventing couple and family discord. Both preventive and treatment programs emphasized education about stepfamilies, suggesting that most stepfamilies need information to normalize their experience and form realistic expectations to successfully adapt to stepfamily life. In addition to normalization, interventions also focus on (1) protecting and strengthening the couples' relationship, focusing on communication and problem-solving skills, (2) appropriate methods of discipline and mutual support between spouses, and (3) dealing with the noncustodial parent. Therapists must keep these considerations in mind when applying evidence-based treatments to couples that are in stepfamilies.

CONCLUSION

Although there's been a strong anti-empirical stance in the history of family therapy (Liddle, 1991; Shields, Wynne, McDaniel, & Gawinski, 1994), a new generation of family therapy students is emerging that are thirsty for scientifically informed strategies. In almost every class we teach, students are asking the question "What does the research say about that treatment approach or intervention in addressing problem X?" Their assumption is that there should be research to support what we do. Although the research on couple and family therapy is far from perfect, there is an enormous amount of evidence supporting the effectiveness of family therapy with a diverse range of clients and problems (Lebow, 2006). In addition, research in family and health sciences illuminates family processes that are harmful and helpful to individual and relational well-being.

Unfortunately, the field of family therapy must also acknowledge the dearth of evidence demonstrating the effectiveness of some beloved models, such as Bowen Theory, and specific interventions, such as externalization. This does not mean that these approaches and interventions are ineffective; however, the evidence supporting their effectiveness is currently lacking. As we have noted throughout the book, no evidence-based treatment will ever extinguish the nuances of clinical practice. But the models we described in this chapter can enhance one's effectiveness and confidence knowing that certain models and strategies carry a seal of approval from quality data.

CHAPTER 17

Apply III

How to Talk to Clients about an Evidence-Based Approach

In earlier chapters we highlighted the therapist's role as a "translator." Another word for the role of the therapist in evidence-based practice (EBP) is the "conductor." A therapist considers the multitude of variables affecting the treatment plan and shares the possibilities with the client. As mentioned in a previous chapter, the client has the right to be informed about the treatment options and to consent (or not) to the treatment plan.

In contrast to historical models where the therapist possessed sole decision-making authority, the EBP model explicitly advocates for **shared decision making**. The therapist presents treatment options based on the best available evidence and then collaborates with the client to determine the best fit given the client's goals, values, and preferences. This step of the EBP process requires that a clinician summarize the results of literature searches in a manner that makes sense to the client, and elicits active participation on the part of the client. Through collaborative dialogue, the therapist and client can arrive at an agreed upon treatment plan.

The wishes of the client in terms of her desire to be involved in treatment decisions should also be considered. Thus, a meta-decision can be made about the process of making treatment decisions when the therapist asks, "How much information would you like me to share about your treatment options?" Increasingly, clients have access to mental health information and want to participate in their care. But at times, clients may still only want a little information and trust the therapist to make most treatment decisions. Still, most of the EBP literature supports shared decision making.

THE SHARED DECISION-MAKING MODEL

Shared decision making is a model of communication between therapists and clients that has been increasingly advocated as an ideal model of treatment because it encourages the respect and autonomy of the patient. Shared decision making is part of a larger social movement in health care that emphasizes a patient-centered approach to treatment instead of the traditional paternalistic approach (Barrett, 2008; Fowler, Levin, & Sepucha, 2011; Légaré et al., 2011; Légaré et al., 2008). The patient-centered approach has been identified as one strategy for improving the quality of health care in America. For instance, in their report on the "quality chasm" in health care in the United States, the Committee on Quality of Health Care in America (2001) identified six core values as the foundation for a better health care system: (1) safe, (2) effective, (3) patient-centered, (4) timely, (5) efficient, and (6) equitable (p. 6). The report states that treatment must be based on the best available scientific evidence, yet customizable to meet the needs and values of different patients. Furthermore, patient preferences should strongly influence health care decisions, and information must be made available to patients and their families so that they can make informed decisions when selecting a treatment option compared to other alternatives.

Charles, Gafni, and Whelan (1997) outline key characteristics that define the shared decision-making model: (1) at least two participants—provider and patient are involved; (2) both parties share information; (3) both parties take steps to build consensus about the goals and preferred treatment; and (4) an agreement is reached on the treatment to implement. The model is seen as an intermediary stage between the paternalistic model, in which the provider dominates the process, and the informed decision-making model, in which the patient assumes sole responsibility for treatment decisions. In this model, the therapist contributes his expertise in evidence-based therapies, while the client contributes her knowledge and experiences that have shaped her personal goals, values, and preferences. Together, the provider and patient consider the treatment options in light of the information exchange and then arrive at a mutually agreed upon treatment approach. Mutual agreement does not mean that both parties are equally convinced that the decided-upon treatment is the best approach overall. Rather, they agree that the plan is the best approach based on their shared deliberation.

SHARED DECISION MAKING IN FAMILY THERAPY

The shared decision-making model has been endorsed by both clients and providers within mental health care (Patel, Bakken, & Ruland, 2008), and it is implicit in both the ethical standards and core competencies set forward by the American Association of Marriage and Family Therapy (AAMFT). For instance, the principle of informed consent implies at least a minimum of shared decision making in the form of information transfer and patient consent to treatment. According to the AAMFT Code of Ethics (2012) 1.2,

> marriage and family therapists obtain appropriate consent to therapy or related procedures as early as feasible in the therapeutic relationship, and use language that is understandable to clients. The content of informed consent may vary depending upon the client and treatment plan; however, informed consent generally necessitates that the client: (a) had the capacity to consent; (b) has been adequately informed of significant information concerning treatment processes and procedures; (c) has been adequately informed of potential risks and benefits of treatments for which generally recognized standards do not yet exist; (d) had freely and with undue influence expressed consent; and (e) has provided consent that is appropriately documented.

Furthermore, according to ethics code 1.8, "marriage and family therapists respect the rights of clients to make decisions and help them understand the consequences of these decisions."

While the AAMFT Code of Ethics' perspective on informed consent can be interpreted in various ways, we believe it highlights the client's active role in treatment decisions. It is the therapist's duty to present information to clients about the nature of treatment, possible alternatives, and potential risks and benefits of various treatment models so that clients can make an informed decision (Fisher & Oransky, 2008). EBP transforms the informed consent process in a way that the therapist is presenting not just his or her preferred approach to treatment, but rather, treatment options based on his or her understanding of the best scientific evidence available.

Furthermore, AAMFT puts forth a set of core competencies for the practice of marriage and family therapy. These competencies are based, in part, on the six core values identified by the Committee on Quality of Health Care in America (Nelson et al., 2007). EBP and the shared decision-making model are evident in several of the competencies required to practice independently as an MFT, including the following:

1. Solicit and use client feedback throughout the therapeutic process (1.3.7).
2. Integrate client feedback, assessment, contextual information, and diagnosis with treatment goals and plan (3.2.1).
3. Comprehend a variety of individual and systemic therapeutic models and their application, including evidence-based therapies and culturally sensitive approaches (4.1.1).
4. Match treatment modalities and techniques to clients' needs, goals, and values (4.3.1).

One major challenge family therapists face when they consider shared decision making is that there is often more than one client. Shared decision making can be more complex when family members have competing views about the best treatment options. Also, family members may have differing views about who the identified patient is and who has the authority to make the treatment decisions. For example, a husband might view his depressed wife as the "problem" and his wife might view the husband's anger as the primary problem. Parents might view their child's poor school performance as the problem that needs treatment. Adult children might view their elderly parents' confusion as the problem, but the elderly parent might want to be left alone. Thus, EBP can be more complex when you are treating a system, not just individuals. In general, the EBP literature is written from a linear perspective. There is one patient who has one or maybe two identifiable and agreed upon diagnoses. The therapist–client dyad makes the decisions.

Another challenge family therapists often face occurs when decision-making authority rests with other family members, and not just the identified patient. For example, adult children might want their elderly parent to consider psychotropic medications, or parents may want their teenage children to participate in an evidence-based treatment for oppositional behavior. At times, the identified client, who will often be the main recipient of treatment, might not agree with the treatment plan. Also, the identified patient may not even be able to give consent to the treatment. For example, children, some disabled adults, and some elderly family members may have only a cursory understanding of their options even when the therapist tries to offer a thoughtful explanation.

Thus, a family therapist has to set the stage for shared treatment planning by making sure to acknowledge each member's particular view of the problem. The therapist needs to recognize the intellectual capacity, interests, and limitations of each family member. Before making treatment decisions, the therapist can help the family members identify a shared goal and hopefully reach some consensus about treatment priorities. Even if most family members agree with the problem definition, if one member disagrees about the problem definition and treatment, the therapy can fail. In contrast, if the therapist respectfully helps the family to reach some consensus about the problem definition, then the stage is set for shared decision making.

THE BENEFITS OF SHARED DECISION MAKING

Shared decision-making not only satisfies the ethical and professional standards for therapists, it also increases the success of treatment outcomes by (1) strengthening the therapeutic relationships, (2) increasing client participation, and (3) helping customize the treatment to the client. The collaborative nature of the shared decision-making process can help to build trust, confidence, and the alliance. The therapeutic relationship or alliance has been shown to account for as much, if not more, of the variance in therapeutic outcomes than the actual approach to treatment or technique (Norcross, 2011). Shared decision making also empowers the client and provides a sense of ownership over the process. Research has demonstrated that treatment adherence and outcomes improve when clients are active participants in the decision-making process (as reviewed in Towle & Godolphin, 1999, and Patel, Bakken, & Ruland, 2008). Furthermore, both collaboration and goal consensus between patient and therapist are associated with better treatment outcomes in the majority of studies reviewed in a recent meta-analysis (Tryon & Winograd, 2011). And finally, critics of evidence-based treatment have often suggested that the EBP model restricts clinical flexibility and dehumanizes clients (e.g., Bohart, O'Hara, & Leitner, 1998; Garfield, 1996). However, the shared decision-making approach helps to fit the evidence-based treatment to the client rather than the other way around. This is a crucial step in more recent models of EBP. If the treatment approach is not compatible with the attitudes and values of the client, then the client is likely to reject the treatment.

WHEN AND HOW MUCH SHOULD YOU EDUCATE CLIENTS ABOUT EBPs?

Involving the family in the shared decision-making process begins with informed consent. Expanding the informed consent process to include a discussion of evidence-based treatments with regard to the patients' characteristics, values, and preferences requires a "process model" rather than an "event model" of informed consent. Several authors have championed this approach to informed consent in psychotherapy (e.g., Pomerantz, 2005; Stone, 1990). They argue that some informed consent topics, such as payment, confidentiality, and supervision are consistent across clients and can be addressed during the first session or shortly thereafter, while other more substantive issues can only take place after a thorough assessment of the presenting problem has occurred. In addition, informed consent is not a one-time event, but an ongoing process throughout the entire therapy. Over time, new concerns may emerge and therapeutic priorities may change. For example, a therapist may initially suggest that medication, psychotherapy, or both are appropriate evidence-based treatments for depression. If the client elects not to pursue medication, the therapist continues to watch and assess the client's symptoms. If the client worsens, the therapist may revisit the treatment options again and perhaps recommend a consultation with a physician or psychiatrist for a medication evaluation while at the same time continuing the evidence-based therapy.

How much information should a therapist actually provide a client about treatment options? It depends upon a number of factors. Legally, a therapist should meet or exceed the typical standard of practice in his community. But this principle is difficult to measure. Another consideration would be what the average client would want to know to help him or her make decisions (Edwards, 2008).

While having informed consumers is generally good and may lead to clients being more participatory in their own care, clinicians should check to make sure that their clients truly understand their options and the possible outcomes of various treatments.

While little research exists regarding how well-informed psychotherapy consumers are about treatment options and outcomes, the issue of consumer knowledge has been addressed in medical literature. For example, Sepucha et al. (2010) found that patients making medical decisions (such as choosing between an operation, a medication, or no treatment at all) may overestimate their own level of understanding. More specifically, they found no significant relationship between how well-informed the patients *felt* and how knowledgeable they actually were. Individuals with less education and of lower socioeconomic status were more likely to overestimate their knowledge than educated, wealthy individuals.

This suggests that physicians and psychotherapists should take extra care in making sure clients understand, even when they say they do. The authors specifically recommend that this can be best accomplished by asking clients specific questions about their care. For example, instead of asking "Do you understand the difference between the treatment options?" a therapist might instead ask a client to explain the difference. This allows the opportunity for further discussion and, if need be, correction. This research also reminds clinicians that not all consumers of psychotherapy will have access to the same knowledge base. Clinicians may need to take special care to explain options and risks to high-risk populations as they are the most vulnerable and the least likely to access such information on their own.

FACTORS INFLUENCING
SHARED DECISION MAKING

Therapists are responsible for informing patients about (1) the potential benefits and risks of treatment, (2) the treatment activities and techniques involved, (3) the number of sessions needed, and (4) the therapist's ability to provide effective treatment. As indicated in the first item, it is important that you consider risks of the treatment, as well as its effectiveness. One has to evaluate the potential harm the treatment could cause a client. For example, most psychotropic drugs have both positive and negative effects. Would your client still be open to taking an antidepressant after learning that it might affect sexual functioning? Often, psychotherapy treatments take longer than psychotropic medications. However, their effects have the potential to be more long-lasting. Some negative effects of psychotropic medications, such as dry mouth or constipation, are also absent in psychotherapy. However, psychotherapy also has the potential to cause harm. The evidence-based literature might not usually address these "risks." Some of these issues could include the cost of the treatment and how that expense would fit into a family's limited budget. It is important that you take this into consideration and discuss this with your client. The literature also might not tell you about other treatment options, especially the treatments that do not have strong empirical support or have yet to be researched. Thus, there are multiple considerations the therapist must keep in mind when sharing decision making with clients.

Clients can actively participate in the process when the therapist solicits their goals, values, and preferences. However, in many cases, clients may not want to be active participants in the decision-making process, which poses a direct challenge to the EBP process. For instance, Arora and McHorney (2000) analyzed data from 2,197 patients from the Medical Outcomes Study and found that 69% of patients preferred to leave the decision-making process up to their medical provider. Patients who were younger, female, had more education, less severe illness, and an active coping style preferred to take a more active role in the decision-making process. Interestingly, clinically depressed patients also endorsed a more active role preference. Another medical study found that most patients prefer to be offered choices, but over half of the patients still chose to leave the final treatment decisions to their providers (Levinson, Kao, Kuby, & Thisted, 2005). Also, about half of the patients preferred to receive treatment information solely from physicians, instead of seeking the information themselves. Like the earlier study, women, highly educated clients, and younger clients were more active in decision making. African American, Hispanic, and elderly clients often wanted their provider to make treatment decisions for them.

Other client factors may also influence the decision-making process. Feeling rushed in the visit or not understanding what the therapist recommends may inhibit the client from active participation. The client's level of motivation and hope for change can facilitate or impede her participation.

A frequently overlooked influence on clients' behaviors is their previous experiences in therapy or friends/family members' experiences and stories about therapy. If a client had a previous therapist who helped them actively participate in decision making and it was a positive therapeutic experience, the client will bring those stories, expectations, and positive sentiments to their new therapy.

Often clients start therapy with some beliefs about the problem definition and vague ideas about what might help. If clients face multiple problems, they may have some ideas about treatment priorities. Also, clients can have beliefs and expectations about the therapist. For example, if a previous client, who offered glowing reviews of the therapist, has referred a friend, the new client may be more willing to engage quickly in the therapeutic process.

Other client characteristics that influence their participation include education level, financial status, insurance, outside demands, and the ability to make independent decisions. For example, a child from an indigent, multi-stressed family will not participate in the same way an educated young adult will. While maintaining the goal of shared decision making, therapists need to tailor their conversations to their specific clients.

Often the clinical context sets the parameters of shared decision making. For example, our students have worked in clinics that use only one clinical model or have specific limits on the types of problems that can be seen or the number of sessions available to clients (often because of funding limits). Other payment systems, including Medicare, Medi-Cal, and private insurance, set specific limits on what are covered benefits. Often, therapeutic resources in a specific community are limited, especially in rural areas. An evidence-based treatment may not be available. A multitude of factors can influence the decision-making process. The more information the therapist has about the context, the better he or she will be in tailoring the treatment recommendations. One of the most common mistakes we have noticed when watching therapists attempt to do EBP practice is their over-focus on a specific treatment model and a disregard for contextual factors that make the model an impractical choice.

HOW TO TALK TO FAMILIES AND LARGER SYSTEMS ABOUT EBP

EBP principles were created using the model of a physician and individual patient making decisions about the patient's health care. Using a simple dyad can make the decision-making process easier than involving multiple stakeholders or clients. As mentioned earlier, treating families can make the decision-making process more complex because every member's perspective has to be considered. This is also true when applying

EBP to other types of systems. For example, some therapists were asked to create a program to treat school bullying. In this case, the therapists had to consider numerous stakeholders in the decision-making process, including school administrators, parents, students, and teachers. In addition, the therapists had to take into account the wishes of the funding organization. When working with multiple stakeholders, the roles, responsibilities, boundaries, and authority lines (hierarchy) have to be considered in the EBP process. Fortunately, family therapists are comfortable working within systems and can incorporate their understanding of how systems operate with the EBP process.

CONCLUSION

Regardless of who the clients or stakeholders are, therapists should incorporate the following steps when talking to their clients:

1. Identify shared goals and hopefully a common definition of the problem. Make sure that every client or stakeholder can give their unique perspective and share their concerns.
2. Summarize the problem list, and decide treatment priorities by again eliciting each client's viewpoint.
3. The therapist can give his initial realistic appraisal of what can be accomplished and what cannot be accomplished given the current circumstances and resources. The therapist also offers to look further into treatment options.
4. Review the literature on options.
5. Summarize your findings to the clients and stakeholders.
6. Lead a discussion about the best path to take. Give your recommendations and explain why you recommend a certain path. Again, make sure each member can give his or her opinion.
7. Reach a consensus on the treatment plan.

Usually this process is fluid and seldom happens in a neat, stepwise progression. It is the caring, concern, and interest of the therapist that makes the EBP treatment recommendations applicable to the hearts and minds of the clients and stakeholders.

CHAPTER 18

Analyze and Adjust

Evaluating Your Clinical Work

Much of this book has been devoted to providing you with a basic overview of research methodology, exposing you to the benefits of evidence-based practice, and highlighting evidenced-based treatment methods that will hopefully be integrated into your work. This chapter asks the following question: How can your research skills help you study your current work with clients? Studying your own practice helps you answer several important questions: How are your clients progressing and what is contributing to their progress (or lack of progress)? Are they getting better, worse, or staying about the same? Can you predict how they'll be doing near the end of therapy? The most treasured treatment models that show so much promise in a research context will have little chance for success if implemented by a therapist who is not keeping track of therapy progress. As we will discuss in this chapter, there's a long, valued history of research that suggests progress in therapy is significantly related to client, therapist, and client–therapist relationship factors. This research supports what advocates of common factors have asserted as critical elements of successful psychotherapy: client motivation, the ability of a therapist to cultivate hope, a strong alliance between therapist and client, a client's expectations that therapy will be helpful, and family alliance (e.g., common understanding, caring, respect for familial bonds) (Chenail et al., 2012).

When we ask our students how they know their therapy is successful, they will often say, "The client attends sessions regularly" or "My client says that he enjoys coming to therapy." Therapy is often deemed as unsuccessful when a client terminates prematurely. Although these conclusions could be accurate, this type of feedback doesn't tell us much about the effectiveness of our work. The client who regularly attends therapy and indicates satisfaction may be making little progress toward her stated goals. Similarly, the client who no shows after several months in therapy and doesn't return to therapy may have benefited significantly from therapy.

When your clients repeatedly complete psychometric instruments, such as the Beck Depression Inventory, Dyadic Adjustment Scale, or PHQ-9, you are tracking their progress in specific areas. What you may not know is how the therapy may or may not be contributing to that change (or lack of change). How satisfied are your clients with you and the therapy? How much does a client trust you? Do you and your client share the same goals? How much progress is being made outside the therapy room? The answers to these questions are often elusive unless we specifically ask.

In this chapter, we will focus on what Howard, Moras, Brill, Martinovich and Lutz (1996) call patient-focused research, or what others have called practice-based evidence (Dattilio et al., 2014). In contrast to treatment-focused research that is concerned with the effectiveness of specific clinical interventions, patient-focused research is concerned with monitoring a client's progress in therapy and using client feedback to inform therapy. Our goal isn't to pit patient-focused research against treatment-focused research. We are in agreement with Norcross and Lambert (2011) who advocate for the synergy of empirically supported relationships and empirically supported treatments to benefit therapists and their clients. Client-focused feedback will allow you to quickly and immediately evaluate the progress of your clinical work, help you understand the change process of your clients, and potentially alter your treatment approach to increase the likelihood of successful outcomes.

EVALUATING THERAPY PROCESS

Therapy process refers to what goes on in the therapy room, particularly the client's experiences in therapy. Several decades of client satisfaction literature has shown that the most helpful aspects of therapy are related to both therapist characteristics and client self-expression. A supportive therapeutic relationship, achieving self-understanding or insight, and the therapist encouraging work outside the therapy (e.g., homework) are also key ingredients to helpful therapy (Elliott & James, 1989).

The current research on therapy process has continued to be robust. The conclusions and recommendations of the second Task Force on Evidence-Based Therapy Relationships confirm what works and doesn't work in clinical practice (Norcross & Wampold, 2011). Helpful processes include the therapy relationship (e.g., alliance between the therapist and client), which we'll discuss in more detail below, the therapist's ability to listen, validate and empathize, collecting client feedback, and goal consensus and general collaboration (Elliot, 2008). Unhelpful processes include therapists being hostile, critical, or blaming, a confrontational style, using assumptions, and therapist rigidity, in terms of the treatment model implemented (e.g., using a treatment model incompatible with the client). A key theme that emerges from these recommendations is the centrality of the therapy relationship.

The therapy relationship, particularly the alliance between the therapist and client, has received much attention in the psychotherapy literature and in clinical training. Alliance, or working alliance, has been defined using three domains (Bordin, 1979): (1) bonds, or trust and respect between a therapist and client; (2) goals, or mutual agreement in achieving certain outcomes; and (3) tasks, or how much the client and therapist agree on certain therapy activities. Developing a working alliance is one of the first skills new therapists learn and try to implement in their work with clients. Therapists intuitively make judgments about their alliance with individual clients. When clients appear motivated, feel understood, and are engaged in the therapy process, it's a sign of progress based on a good therapeutic relationship. When clients seem disinterested, angry, or misunderstood, an assumption might be made that joining hasn't yet occurred and the therapeutic relationship needs to be strengthened.

When working with couples and families, the therapist–client alliance becomes exponentially more complicated. Multiple alliances exist and interact with one another in a circular fashion. In couple therapy, for example, one isn't simply adding another person and alliance to the therapy room. A therapist's empathic statement to a wife may be perceived negatively by the husband, which might strengthen the therapist–wife alliance and weaken the therapist–husband alliance. The therapist is frequently negotiating contrasting goals for therapy and varying levels of motivation from individual family members.

Accessing the client's impression of therapy alliance is not just important for greater retention; it also strongly influences the course of treat-ment. Research has repeatedly found that alliance between the therapist and family members is consistently related to better therapy outcomes and is a key ingredient to client change (Diamond, Liddle, Hogue, & Dakof, 1999; Heatherington & Friedlander, 1990; Johnson, Wright, & Ketring, 2002; Robbins et al., 2008; Shirk & Karver, 2003). Although a strong alliance doesn't guarantee a successful outcome, a poor alliance is highly predictive of a poor outcome. Improving a poor alliance is critical in achieving a better outcome (Miller, Duncan, Brown, Sorrell, & Chalk, 2006). Friedlander et al. (2006) recommend periodically asking clients to complete a brief measure of the alliance, which provides an opportu-nity for therapists to directly address and repair problematic alliances. A few of the most widely used self-report measures of therapy alliance are described next.

The *Session Rating Scale* (SRS; Duncan & Miller, 2008) is a four-item pencil-and-paper scale designed to assess key dimensions of effective therapeutic relationships or therapy alliance. Metaphorically, it takes the temperature of the session. At the end of the session, a therapist can ask a client to complete the SRS to evaluate the session, with a particu-lar focus on the effectiveness of the therapist: Did the client feel heard, understood, and respected by the therapist? Did the therapist focus on areas the client wanted to work on and talk about? Was the therapist's approach a good fit for the client? Finally, did the overall session feel right or was something missing? The therapist can review the results with the client at the end of the session, or review it between sessions and discuss the data at the next session.

The *Working Alliance Inventory* (WAI; Horvath & Greenberg, 1986, 1989) measures Bordin's three aspects of the alliance described earlier in this chapter: (1) the bond ("I feel comfortable with _____"); (2) the agreement on goals ("I wish _____ and I could clarify the goals of our sessions"); and (3) the agreement on tasks ("We agree on what is important for me to work on"). The WAI is a 36-item ques-tionnaire with 12 items for each dimension of Bordin's alliance concept. Each item is rated on a 7-point scale (1 = never, 7 = always). Shortened versions of the WAI have been developed (see Hatcher & Gillaspy, 2006; Tracey & Kokotovic, 1989). Research has shown support for the reliabil-ity and validity of the WAI (Horvath, 1994).

The *Couple Therapy Alliance Scale* (CTAS) and *Family Therapy Alliance Scale* (FTAS) stem from Pinsof and Catherall's (1986) inte-grative psychotherapy alliance model and encompass four domains: (1)

self–therapist targets the alliance (tasks, goals, and bonds) between the therapist and the client (e.g., "The therapist and me . . . "); (2) other–therapist addresses the client's perception of the alliance between the therapist and other family member(s) (e.g., "The therapist and my partner . . . "); (3) group–therapist focuses on the client's perception of the alliance between the client's family, including the client, and the therapist (e.g., "The therapist and us . . . "); and (4) within-system refers to the client's perception of the alliance between the client and the people who are important to her or him (e.g., "My partner and I . . . "), but does not include the therapist. The FTAS and CTAS each contain 29 items. Both are rated on a 7-point Likert-type scale with responses ranging from completely disagree (1) to completely agree (7).

The *Vanderbilt Therapeutic Alliance Scale* (VTAS; Hartley & Strupp, 1983) identifies aspects of the relationship between individual family members and the therapist in the context of family sessions. Ratings are based on observations of family members' behaviors and therapist–family member interactions as they occur in the sessions. Twenty-six items are rated on a Likert-type scale ranging from 0 (not at all) to 5 (a great deal). A revised, pared down version was created in 1996 (Shelef & Diamond, 2008). Unlike the other scales, the VTAS and VTAS-r are observer-based scales, meaning a rater observes and codes a therapy session. The VTAS would be most useful in a training context, where time and resources are greater and information can be reported back to therapists in training.

The *System for Observing Family Therapy Alliances* (SOFTA; Friedlander et al., 2006) looks at four alliance dimensions: (1) Safety within the Therapeutic System measures each client's degree of comfort taking risks, being vulnerable, and exploring conflicts with a therapist and other family members; (2) Engagement in the Therapeutic Process measures agreement with the therapist on tasks and goals; (3) Emotional Connection with the Therapist measures the therapist–client bond; and 4) Shared Sense of Purpose within the Family refers to productive family collaboration (the within-family alliance). SOFTA is also published in a Spanish version, *Sistema de la Observación de la Alianza en Terapia Familiar.*

EVALUATING THERAPY OUTCOMES

Outcome research refers to whether the client is experiencing change. More specifically, it examines whether the client is benefiting from therapy. Kenneth Howard is a pioneer in outcome research, particularly through his dosage model of psychotherapeutic effectiveness (Howard, Kopte, Krause & Orlinsky, 1986; Howard, Lueger, Maling, & Martinovich, 1993; Howard et al., 1996). His research exposed the relationship between the number of sessions and probability of client improvement (e.g., most change takes places earlier in treatment rather than later), and articulated three phases of treatment: (1) remoralization (giving clients hope when they feel demoralized); (2) remediation (bring relief of client's symptoms); and (3) rehabilitation (unlearning maladaptive coping strategies). Howard's research helped make the therapy process more transparent, which provided a window into client change and sparked other groundbreaking research in this area (Lebow, 2006).

Lambert et al. (2001) determined when client-focused feedback was provided to therapists, alerting them of potential treatment failure with at-risk clients, outcomes improved. The idea of client-focused feedback is consistent with Howard's idea of measuring how clients are doing while we're working with them in order to tailor our work to their needs. We can continue what's working well and modify our approach when treatment is stagnant or potentially making things worse.

How does a therapist receive client-focused feedback? Standardized scales can be used to track client change. The data is immediately available to clinicians. Lambert and Shimokawa (2011) explain the basic rationale behind collecting client feedback:

> If we get information about what seems to be working, and more importantly what is not working, our responsiveness to clients will improve. In many situations, performance and feedback are intertwined and obvious; in others, a certain degree of blinding occurs, such that the association is not so temporally connected and the effects of performance are harder to discern (such as in psychotherapy), making it much more difficult for the therapist to learn and improve. (p. 72)

Some therapists have an overly optimistic view of client progress, overlook negative changes, and are not particularly successful at predicting treatment outcome (Lambert & Shimokawa, 2011). These trends that mostly come from research with experienced therapists in private practice and advanced students may not be consistent for beginning master's therapists, who tend to be overly self-critical and sometimes perseverate on negative changes. However, the research in this area is making an important point: Therapists often don't *really* know how their clients are progressing; it's often left to intuition. Data helps makes therapy progress more transparent.

Michael Lambert at Brigham Young University and his colleagues have done extensive research on tracking client outcomes in psychotherapy. They developed the OQ-A, a computer-based feedback system for monitoring and enhancing treatment effectiveness. The system helps therapists determine if their clients are staying on track toward positive treatment outcomes and helps them get their clients back on track if treatment is not progressing effectively. The implementation of the system is modified depending on the progress of the client. Part of the system is only used when clients are showing a lack of progress in therapy.

The *Outcome Questionnaire–45* (OQ-45; Lambert et al., 2004) is a 45-item self-report measure for adult clients that can be given at the beginning of sessions and at termination. The system is set up to be computer-based in order to generate reports for the therapist, but you could use a hardcopy version to simplify. It measures three areas of client functioning: (1) symptoms of psychological disturbance; (2) interpersonal problems; and (3) social role functioning. Higher scores suggest greater levels of disturbance. While therapists can access similar information with other assessment instruments like the Beck Depression Inventory, the PHQ-9, the Family Assessment Device, and/or the Dyadic Adjustment Scale, the OQ-45 allows therapists to assess multiple areas with one questionnaire. Repeated administration allows therapists to track change over time. The results provide a "mental health vital sign," including the ability to predict treatment failure based on pretreatment distress scores (Lambert & Shimokawa, 2011).

A child and youth version, the *Youth Outcome Questionnaire* (Y-OQ), is also available. The Y-OQ is a 64-item instrument completed by the parent or guardian as a measure of treatment progress for children and youth ages 4–17 (Burlingame, Wells, Lambert, & Cox, 2004). The 64 items include six separate subscales: interpersonal distress, somatic, interpersonal relationships, critical items, social problems, and behavioral dysfunction. The primary goal of the Y-OQ is to track changes in functioning.

After clients complete the OQ-45 or Y-OQ, they may be prompted to complete another questionnaire, the *Assessment for Signal Cases* (ASC; Lambert et al., 2007), if they are not making expected gains and are at risk for a poor outcome. The ASC is a 40-item measure that generates data about problems in the therapy when a client is not making progress or is worsening. The ASC measures therapy alliance, negative life events, social support outside of therapy, and motivation. The ASC directs a therapist's attention to problematic areas to help make necessary treatment decisions. For example, a medication referral may be necessary if the client is working hard in therapy but getting worse. Or, the therapist might learn that she needs to use a more structured form of therapy (Rousmaniere, 2013).

Similar to Lambert and his colleagues, Scott Miller, Barry Duncan, and their colleagues have been advocating for therapist knowledge about progress in therapy. Rather than guessing that therapy is effective, they've been encouraging therapists to measure outcomes from session to session by using standardized outcomes measurement tools to learn what's working and not working in therapy (Duncan, Miller, & Sparks, 2004). Their concerns about the time commitment in completing and analyzing the most frequently used instruments led them to create brief instruments that could be quickly completed, analyzed, and discussed with clients.

Miller, Duncan, Sorrell, and Brown's (2005) *Partners for Change Outcome Management System* (PCOMS) includes two brief scales (four items each) that a client completes and reviews with the therapist during the session. *The Session Rating Scale* (SRS) was described in our earlier discussion about alliance. *The Outcome Rating Scale* (ORS; Miller, Duncan, Brown, Sparks, & Claud, 2003) is a four-item scale designed to assess areas of life functioning known to change as a result of therapeutic intervention. At the beginning of the session, a client is asked to quietly complete the ORS, which gives a snapshot of how the client is doing on a scale of 1–10 at that moment in time in three areas over the past week: individually, interpersonally (family), and socially (work, school, friendships). In addition, the client is asked to evaluate how he or she is doing overall (general well-being). The scale is scored immediately. Once a score is determined, the score can be easily placed on a graph to track progress from session to session. When the therapist and client are able to see which of the three areas receives the lowest scores, it can sometimes help determine areas that need immediate attention.

In comparison to Lambert's Q-A computer-based system, the ORS doesn't provide as much detailed information about a client's functioning. However, the simplicity and brevity of the instrument and the ability to process the information in session with the client increases the likelihood that therapists will integrate client feedback into their work. The ORS, along with the SRS, are available in multiple languages at *http:// scottdmiller.com/performance-metrics*.

CASE EXAMPLE

The following case illustrates how one therapist integrated the ORS into her work with a couple. Allen, a 69-year-old veteran, came to therapy with his wife, Frances, who was 63 and also a veteran. The couple was referred to therapy by Allen's individual therapist because Allen complained his wife seemed unhappy in the marriage. He expressed confusion as to why she was unhappy, and indicated that he was content in the marriage. At the beginning of the second session, the therapist (Mandy) gave both partners the ORS to complete. The different levels of satisfaction with the marriage were clearly evident on the ORS. On the interpersonal scale, Allen scored a 9.5 while Frances scored a 2.5.

Mandy continued to have Allen and Frances take a couple of minutes at the beginning of each session to complete the ORS. She found this helpful in tracking how things were going in their individual lives and in their relationship. The ORS scores for both partners plotted over time (see Figure 18.1) reflected what happened over the course of therapy. As Frances began to express her dissatisfactions with the marriage and request changes in therapy, Allen would become upset. Not surprisingly, his scores on the interpersonal scale dipped as the initial work of therapy began. While Mandy encouraged Frances to articulate her concerns so that things could improve, she also tried to support Allen by acknowledging how difficult it must be to hear how unhappy his wife was with him. Mandy helped the couple negotiate some behavioral changes that Frances requested, which Allen was willing and capable of doing (e.g., more participation in household chores). As Allen made these changes, Frances's scores on the interpersonal and overall scales improved dramatically. Allen's scores on the interpersonal scale did not rebound initially, but his scores eventually returned to their initially high level once he grew accustomed to the new responsibilities and saw how much happier his wife was with the changes that had been made. Allen liked that Frances had become much less irritable with him.

Mandy also found the ORS scores helpful in monitoring how stressful events in Allen's life were impacting him. On the initial ORS, Mandy noted that Allen scored a 1.5 on the social scale, which he attributed to stressors he was experiencing in his volunteer work where he had primary responsibility for an upcoming event. Successfully getting through this event and retiring from this volunteer position eventually led to improvement in his social scale scores. Stress in this and other areas led to many ups and downs in terms of Allen's well-being scores. A health scare in the

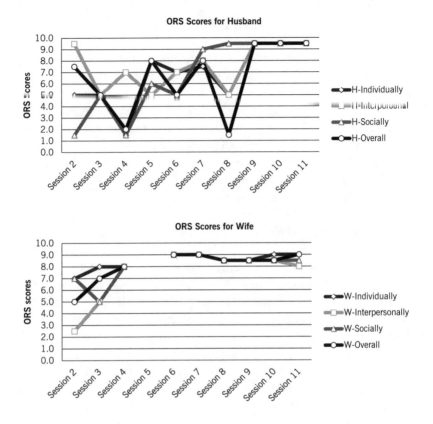

FIGURE 18.1. Outcome Rating Scale (ORS) scores for a couple.

week prior to the eighth session resulted in Allen's overall score dipping to a low of 1.5. Thankfully the health issue was resolved, and his scores rebounded. A portion of therapy was devoted to discussing these stressful events in his life, including one individual session when Frances was out of town. This helped Allen feel supported by the therapist. In addition, it was indirectly beneficial to Frances, who reported that his stress negatively impacted her because she would worry about him.

CLIENT-FOCUSED PROGRESS RESEARCH FOR FAMILY THERAPISTS

To this point, much of the client-focused feedback we've discussed has been mostly relevant for individual therapy. Although the measures described above can be applied to family therapy work as shown in the example above, William Pinsof and his colleagues specifically designed the *Systemic Therapy Inventory of Change* (STIC) to help therapists who work with couples and families (Breunlin, Pinsof, & Russell, 2011; Pinsof et al., 2009). The STIC is the first measurement system designed to track change in family and couple therapy and has five scales for assessing five areas in a family system: Individual Problems and Strengths, Family of Origin, Relationship with Partner, Family/Household, and Child Problems and Strengths (Pinsof et al., 2009). It generates self-report, web-based feedback about initial client concerns, tracks change from session to session, and provides information about the therapeutic alliance over the course of therapy.

The measurement system has three distinct instruments: (1) The Initial STIC, which is a lengthy instrument administered to clients before the beginning of therapy, including demographic information; (2) the Intersession STIC, which is a much briefer instrument given to clients before each session; and (3) the Short Form Integrative Psychotherapy Alliance Scales, which are administered along with the Intersession STIC. Friedlander (2009) describes the power of the STIC:

> The beauty of the system is that it allows predictions to be tested about how change in one domain may be related to change in another. Does a decrease in couples' conflict, for example, predict improved child behavior, even when only the partners take part in treatment? (p.130)

The STIC can test a multitude of other hypotheses: Does a reduction in depressive symptoms help reduce marital distress? Does a strong therapy alliance with an adolescent girl help facilitate change between the adolescent and her mother? Does therapy with a particular part of the family, or the use of a particular model of therapy (e.g., narrative therapy), have an impact on change in the family? STIC data are stored on a secure website and includes bar graphs with initial scores and change profiles on the scales over the course of therapy. Therapists can view the data prior to a session and also review the data with clients during a session.

There are valid concerns about using an instrument like the STIC, such as the time commitment for completion between sessions for therapists and clients. How can therapists and clients stay committed to the system over time? A bigger concern for independent practitioners is the financial cost associated with purchasing and maintaining the system. Eventually, the STIC, or data systems like the STIC, will be readily accessible and affordable. Currently, the Family Institute at Northwestern is offering the STIC at a nominal cost to all mental health training programs. For programs interested in a valid feedback mechanism, the STIC would be an invaluable training tool to give trainees immediate feedback on their progress with couples and families, which could be brought into clinical supervision for review and discussion.

CONCLUSION

In this chapter, we have reviewed a range of instruments that provide feedback to therapists to monitor a client or family's response to therapy and satisfaction with the therapy relationship. Research has shown that this kind of feedback to therapists likely improves outcomes, particularly for clients at risk for therapy dropout (Lambert & Shimokawa, 2011). Although some of these tools are lengthy and costly (e.g., OQ; STIC), they provide a wealth of information at the beginning of treatment and enable a therapist to clearly track progress over time. Other tools (e.g., ORS, SRS) are quite brief and take only a few minutes to complete in session; these tools can be integrated into one's work immediately.

CHAPTER 19

The Future
of Evidence-Based Practice

Looking into the Crystal Ball

Health care reform in the United States means that more patients will have access to mental health care (Lubell, 2013). A law requiring that mental health benefits are commensurate with physical benefits and laws requiring a minimal benefits mandate provide mental health and substance abuse coverage to more than 32 million Americans who did not have mental health benefits before. Under these new guidelines, treatments are expected to be supported by empirical research. Thus, evidence-based practice (EBP) has become a major influence on how health care is delivered, and is now considered a means of ensuring accountability within the health care system (Crane & Hafen, 2002).

Support for EBP in federal policy reflects the culmination of health care professionals' efforts to identify optimal patient care. Beginning early in the 20th century, physicians and epidemiologists in both the United States and the United Kingdom pushed for treatments that were empirically supported, attempting to hold physicians accountable and provide the best care possible (Spring, 2007). As mentioned in earlier chapters, multiple initiatives in many countries coalesced in Canada during the 1980s and 1990s when the McMaster group developed a system to help physicians use research evidence in their medical practices (Oxman, Sackett, & Guyatt, 1993). Later, these ideas were adopted by many others, including mental health professionals.

While all mental health professions have shifted toward a paradigm that incorporates elements of EBP, some fields have made the transition more quickly and to a greater extent than others. Since some family therapists have little research training, they may be more reluctant to incorporate EBPs (Karam & Sprenkle, 2010). Historically, family therapists focused on the "art" of psychotherapy and placed less emphasis on using science for research-informed care (Hodgson, Johnson, Ketring, Wampler, & Lamson, 2005; Patterson et al., 2004). More recently, all mental health fields, including family therapists, have recognized the growing influence of the EBP movement.

While there have been large differences among family therapists in the application of research to inform their work, the gap is lessening. In the early 2000s, there was an increase in the number of articles published on the efficacy of family therapy models (Patterson et al., 2004). Furthermore in 2002, the American Association for Marriage and Family Therapy (AAMFT) published a book that included several reviews of family therapy literature (Sprenkle, 2004), which were also published in the *Journal of Marital and Family Therapy* (JMFT). In 2012, a special issue (Volume 38, Issue 1) of JMFT provided updated reviews of the family therapy literature. In recent years, a number of articles have been published in JMFT that urge family therapists to incorporate research into their practices (Hodgson et al., 2005; Karam & Sprenkle, 2010; Patterson et al., 2004; Williams et al., 2006). In addition, family-based research is published in periodicals such as the *Journal of Family Psychology, The American Journal of Family Therapy,* and *Family Process,* among others.

EBP will certainly continue to evolve in the years to come and increasingly, payment systems will be tied to EBP. This chapter highlights some of the growing influences of the EBP movement on mental health service delivery. Though no one can predict the future with certainty, it seems that the EBP movement is quickly gaining support in a number of fields, including those that historically do not prioritize research. As the EBP movement continues to gain momentum, it will likely become an even greater priority among payers, government leaders, educators, professional organizations, and consumers of mental health services.

THE INFLUENCE
OF THE FEDERAL GOVERNMENT

While medical educators are given credit for creating the EBP movement, in recent years, payers and policy experts have promoted its growth and influence (Edwards, Patterson, Vakili, & Scherger, 2012). The Affordable Care Act, a U.S. government initiative to increase the number of Americans who have health insurance, mentions evidence-based practice 47 times (University of Georgia, Institute for Evidence-Based Health Profession Education, 2012). While the Affordable Care Act promotes EBP, reviewers have also noted that it does not include funding to support its EBP aims. Nevertheless, a multitude of government agencies are focusing their efforts on supporting EBP.

Funding Research in General

One of the primary ways the government will shape the future of EBP is by funding research. Through funded research on mental health, clinicians will have access to a broader range of evidence to incorporate into their work. For example, the government funds the National Institute of Mental Health (NIMH). While all research has the potential to be helpful, NIMH specifically addresses clinicians' need for support in applying research. This priority is reflected in NIMH's spending. In 2012, NIMH reported spending $174.064 million on research that was specifically geared toward helping community therapists use evidence-based treatments (National Institute of Mental Health, 2012). Other government agencies, such as the National Institute of Health (NIH), the National Institute on Drug Abuse (NIDA), and the Substance Abuse and Mental Health Services Administration (SAMSHA), also support research that can be used by therapists. In addition, local and state governments sometimes fund research and evaluation of mental health initiatives.

Government Agencies and Initiatives for Improving Health Care

While federal funding certainly has a large impact on the state of mental health services and the amount of information that clinicians can draw upon, the government also shapes EBP by creating organizations specifically devoted to improving health care. A specific example of this is the Agency for Healthcare Research and Quality (AHRQ; *www.ahrq.gov*), a government agency devoted to improving health care through the creation of evidence-based practice centers (EPCs). EPCs are public or private organizations that receive funding from the AHRQ in order to generate systematic reviews of the scientific literature. EPCs publish reports of their findings so that health care professionals can quickly and easily access a wealth of vetted research and utilize this knowledge in their practice (Agency for Healthcare Research and Quality, 2011). By generating these reports, the EPCs put research in a format that is digestible for those individuals who do not have research training. Another group affiliated with the AHRQ that supports EBPs is the United States Preventive Services Task Force (USPSTF; *www.ahrq.gov/clinic/uspstfix.htm*). The mission of USPSTF is to make evidence-based recommendations about clinical preventive services.

Government leaders recognize that it is not enough to fund research and hope that practitioners use the research evidence. They go further by evaluating the evidence and providing specific treatment recommendations based on the evidence. For example, in making its recommendations, the USPSTF will "grade" the evidence in terms of its quality and the strength of specific research findings. Thus, the typical clinician can read a few sentences about how to treat a problem and also have some assurance that the treatment is effective.

Given that many practitioners struggle with translating scientific evidence into action, the AHRQ also developed an initiative called Translating Research into Practice (TRIP-II). TRIP-II focuses on evaluating EBP training programs, learning how practitioners go about finding and implementing research. TRIP-II also evaluates which factors influence how successful clinicians are at implementing research into their practice (Agency for Healthcare Research and Quality, 2001). Like EPCs, TRIP-II publishes concise reports of their findings. This means that clinicians and organizations that are interested in applying research, but are uncertain about how to do so, can look at TRIP-II research to learn the most effective strategies. While the current USPSTF, EPC, and TRIP-II databases primarily have information regarding medical issues (diabetes, heart disease, etc.), it is likely that they will expand to include behavioral and mental health issues in the future.

Beyond the Federal Government: Global Initiatives

This section has emphasized the influence of the federal government on EBP. In the future, we may also see international organizations play an important role in developing and disseminating EBP guidelines. For example, the World Health Organization (2010) created the *mhGAP Intervention Guide* to address global mental health issues (*http://whqlibdoc. who.int/publications/2010/9789241548069_eng.pdf*). The guide is intended to help health care professionals in nonspecialized health settings address mental, neurological, and substance abuse disorders they may encounter.

Assessment and treatment recommendations were developed based on systematic reviews by international experts, along with reviewers across the world.

PAY-FOR-PERFORMANCE INCENTIVES

The government and other organizations, such as health insurance companies, have attempted to improve health care outcomes by using payments called "pay-for-performance incentives," also known as **P4P**. Ideally, P4P incentive programs work by measuring a broad range of outcome variables (e.g., patient satisfaction, continuity of care, change in patient distress before and after treatment) for a group of health care providers (Eijkenaar, 2013). If a group of providers reaches optimum performance levels, as specified by a particular P4P program, then the group receives a cash incentive (Agency for Healthcare Research and Quality, 2012). In theory, this automatically prompts providers to look at the research, so that they might know the best treatment available. It also encourages them to examine their own practices, question their own effectiveness, and adjust accordingly. In short, P4P programs attempt to promote EBP.

P4P programs have almost exclusively focused on physicians and physical health care (Bremer, Scholle, Keyser, Knox Houtsinger, & Pincus, 2008). However, there is a possibility of applying P4P in behavioral health care as well (Bremer et al., 2008). For example, physicians have been increasingly incentivized to screen for depression. In some practices, all patients are required to complete the PHQ-2, which is a two-item instrument that assesses if the patient has experienced little interest or pleasure in doing things over the past 2 weeks, or if they report feeling down, depressed, or hopeless (Rosser, Frede, Conrad, & Heaton, 2003). If the responses hit a certain threshold, the patients are then given the full PHQ-9, which is a more thorough screening device. If someone screens positive for depression on the PHQ-9, the provider is expected to address the patient's depressive symptoms regardless of what their primary complaint is (Kroenke, Spitzer, & Williams, 2001). Depression is just one area where physicians are incentivized to address mental health issues.

AHRQ and other groups have funded research on P4P programs to determine whether they actually work (Agency for Healthcare Research and Quality, 2012). So far, the results are mixed and there is much debate about their effectiveness (Rosenthal & Frank, 2006). It is unclear how large of a role P4P programs will play in the future of EBP, but they do have the potential to bolster the movement's momentum.

MINING ELECTRONIC MEDICAL RECORDS FOR TRENDS AND EVIDENCE

Another initiative the government supports is increased use of the electronic medical record (EMR). Government leaders and health researchers recognize that EMRs can be mined to easily collect data on health trends. For example, using data mined from search engines, scientists have detected evidence of unreported drug side effects when patients take both an antidepressant and another common medication. This negative drug interaction was found before it was identified by the usual government warning systems (Markoff, 2013). In addition, the EMR provides an easy way to share information. Both of these traits can strengthen implementation of EBPs. In fact, some advocates of the EMR suggest that in the future, EBP treatment findings and recommendations could "pop up" when a provider writes certain trigger words such as depression or chronic pain. Family therapists will need to become proficient using the EMR if they are going to stay abreast of trends in EBP (Edwards, Patterson, Scherger, & Valiki, in press). Systems have received funding and other types of support to switch from paper files to EMRs.

THE INFLUENCE OF PAYERS

In addition to the federal government's regulations and incentives to provide evidence-based care, we must also consider that therapy is a business. For individual clinicians, providing psychotherapy may be a humanitarian pursuit. However, it is also a multi-million-dollar industry. While there will always be clients who pay out-of-pocket for their treatment, the majority of psychotherapy consumers do not pay for their care. Psychotherapy is generally paid for by insurance companies or by county, state, or federal funding. While clinicians and clients may or may not be concerned with EBP, many of these third-party agencies are insisting upon use of empirically supported treatments (Levant & Hasan, 2008). In fact, this trend is so strong that some prominent mental health care providers have predicted that third-party payers will eventually stop reimbursing clinicians for services that are not supported by research (Cummings, 2006). If this were to happen, it would force clinicians to either adopt EBP or find a way to work outside of managed care by only accepting clients who pay out-of-pocket (Thomason, 2010). Furthermore, the prevalence of EBP may cause professional liability insurance providers to question the use of any therapies not supported by research (Thomason, 2010). While a policy like this may seem extreme since not all valuable therapies have been studied rigorously, it is important that clinicians recognize the requirements that third-party payers might place upon clinicians in the future. Also, therapists who work as part of a **patient centered medical home** (PCMH) team or within an integrated health care system will be required to use EBP treatments (Edwards et al., 2012). The concept of a PCMH was created to improve primary care as part of the U.S. government's health care reform initiatives. Standards suggest that care should be organized around patients' needs. Also, working in teams, coordinating care, and tracking progress over time are all important parts of the PCMH.

THE ROLE OF EDUCATORS

Deficits in Training and Education

Despite the importance of clinical work being informed by research, it seems that many mental health professionals are just now learning how to integrate research findings into their practice. For example, a survey of doctoral students in clinical psychology programs found that most students were unable to explain the essential components of EBP and ranked research as one of their lowest priorities when formulating treatment plans. This is not to say that students do not desire such knowledge. In fact, the same study also found that students wanted further training in EBP (Luebbe, Radcliffe, Callands, Green, & Thorn, 2007). These findings may be replicated among students in other professions. There also may be individual differences in how eager students are to learn more about EBP and to adopt research-informed practice regardless of their professional identities.

Misunderstanding and undervaluing EBP is not limited to students. Nelson and Graves (2011) surveyed 138 AAMFT-approved supervisors and found that of all the 128 core competencies listed by AAMFT, supervisors ranked the ability to critically evaluate research as the 123rd most important skill for supervisees to master. This suggests that some supervisors may place a low priority on their supervisees' ability to deliver research-informed care. Furthermore, supervisors reported that when they did consider their supervisees' ability to deliver research-informed care, the supervisees generally fell short of their supervisors' expectations. This suggests that training in EBP may be lacking during internship years as well as in graduate programs.

Unless professors and supervisors make EBP a priority, it is unlikely that the next generation of therapists will value, understand, or be skilled in delivering EBP. Such a transition will be an emerging shift in clinical education. While a paradigm shift of this magnitude will certainly take time, some proponents of EBP have already published guides that clearly outline different ways to incorporate EBP while still maintaining an emphasis on clinical practice (Beidas, Koerner, Weingardt, & Kendall, 2011; Karam & Sprenkle, 2010; Lebow, 2006; Leffler, Jackson, West, McCarty, & Atkins, 2012; Williams et al., 2006). In a nutshell, educators are encouraged to help students use EBP principles when students are searching for ways to help their clients. Students will be most motivated to learn EBP when the EBP skills help them with their own clients. In addition, clinical programs that primarily train clinicians, not researchers, might want to change their research class to a focus on training therapists to be "research users and appreciators." As these ideas are further developed and integrated, therapists of the future will likely value research and feel comfortable using it to inform their clinical work. In addition, students will be exposed to needed skills for implementation of EBP information. These skills include familiarity with the electronic medical record, team-based interdisciplinary care, screening tools for assessment, data management of client's progress on clinical indicators such as the PHQ-9 for depression, and evidence-based databases accessible on the web (Edwards et al., 2012).

How Research Can Inform EBP Education

In order for clinicians to feel comfortable and confident incorporating research findings into their work, educators will need to bridge gaps that have existed for decades. Though the process may take time and will certainly pose some challenges, continued research can guide educators as to where they might focus their attention. Current research is looking into the common obstacles that professionals may face when attempting to adopt EBP as well as some of the most-effective ways of teaching EBP. By utilizing research on psychotherapy education programs and EBP to inform their pedagogy, educators can anticipate some of the obstacles they might face in trying to teach the principles of EBP.

For example, Bauer (2007) suggests that EBP might be best advanced by not only teaching students *about* EBP, but also by giving them experiential learning opportunities where they will actually need to implement the knowledge they have gained. For example, educators might show their students a video of a therapy session or offer them a vignette and then ask students to find research that is relevant to that particular case. Instead of stopping there, educators might also have students develop a treatment plan based upon the research they found, the characteristics of the client, and their own clinical expertise or intuition. Such a task not only teaches students about EBP, but also allows them to actually utilize EBP. By seeking out articles on implementing EBP, educators might have better EBP learning outcomes.

This idea is supported by literature reviews on the most-effective ways of training therapists. For example, Herschell, Kolko, Baumann, and Davis (2010) reviewed 55 studies that evaluated the utility of six different strategies for training therapists in psychotherapy skills. They found that some of the most-common methods of teaching, such as reading manuals, self-directed trainings (i.e., videos, computer-assisted training programs), and workshops, do not generally result in sustained learning outcomes. While these methods did increase therapists' knowledge, they often failed to result in behavior change (i.e., therapists were not *applying* the knowledge they gained). However, the authors were able to identify some methods of instruction that did result in sustained change: supervision, consultation, feedback following experiential learning, and multicomponent training packages (trainings that involve a combination of manuals, workshops, consultation, and experiential learning opportunities). Furthermore, the authors report that workshops can be highly effective if followed up with additional trainings or if preceded by other methods of instruction. This is unfortunately not a common practice.

While these methods require more time and resources, the literature suggests that they are the most-effective methods of training therapists. This appears to be the case regardless of whether therapists are learning to conduct a particular type of therapy, such as dialectical behavior therapy, or something broad, such as learning to apply research in clinical practice. Other authors (Beidas & Kendall, 2010; Leffler et al., 2012) have reported similar findings and suggestions: teaching EBP should be done in ways that are supported by research and currently, it appears that the most-effective teaching strategies are those that involve active learning. By drawing upon this literature, educators from both clinical and scientist–practitioner models are more likely to have competent and confident students who go on to deliver EBP.

It is important to note, however, that the training method is not the only factor determining whether therapists can or will utilize EBP. There are individual therapist characteristics (such as motivation) as well as organizational factors (such as resources) that still need to be researched further (Herschell et al., 2010). In fact, these issues are so complex that there is an entire literature base developing in translational and implementation science which explores how organizations can implement EBP. Translational science was introduced earlier in the book (Chapter 15). At times, health professionals have used "translational" and "implementation" interchangeably. But, translational has a broader meaning that includes "harnessing basic science to produce new drugs, devices and treatment options for patients" (Woolf, 2008, p. 211). It also includes what is usually referred to as implementation science, which refers to "translating research into practice; i.e., ensuring that new treatments . . . actually reach the patients . . . for whom they are intended and are implemented correctly (Woolf, 2008, p. 211). Steven Woolf (2008) provides an excellent article articulating the meaning of translational and implementation sciences. Other literature describing clinical application of evidence includes Aarons, Hulburt, and McCue-Horwitz (2011) and Damschroder et al. (2009).

Research can also inform training methods by targeting specific learning obstacles. For example, Pagoto et al. (2007) found that misconceptions about EBP were a common barrier to professionals' ability to implement EBP. This suggests that educators may need to pay special attention to debunking common misconceptions about EBP. For example, students may believe that being research-informed requires a deep understanding of advanced statistics or that EBP means adhering to highly structured and manualized treatments. As researchers learn more about successful EBP education, educators will be able to develop ways to better support students as they learn the principles of EBP.

THE ROLE
OF PROFESSIONAL ORGANIZATIONS

EBP skills and research findings will be disseminated by professional organizations that wish to support clinicians who are seeking to expand their skill set to include EBP. Many mental health professional organizations include both researchers and clinicians in order to help members integrate their unique expertise within a scientific forum so that they can translate knowledge into better public policies and clinical practice. Most professional associations require EBP to be addressed in training curriculums. They also offer professional journals, clinical updates, podcasts, online training sites and workshops to help their members learn about EBP and stay abreast of emerging trends.

The American Psychological Association (APA) is also playing an active role in shaping the future of EBP. In 1995, the APA advanced EBP by pushing for evidence-based treatments. While this created controversy over the role of manualized treatments, it ultimately pushed the field toward a model in which clinicians would use their clinical experience, research findings, and the characteristics of the client to inform clinical decisions (Satterfield et al., 2010). Since then, the APA has continued to help clinicians to adopt EBP by doing the following:

1. Developing committees whose job is to examine research and make recommendations for evidence-based treatment methods (Kurtzman & Bufka, 2011).
2. Forming councils whose job is to come up with new ways of supporting clinicians who wish to learn and implement EBP principles (American Psychological Association, 2012a).
3. Publishing policy statements regarding EBP (American Psychological Association, 2005).
4. Offering courses designed to help clinicians understand and adopt EBP (American Psychological Association, 2012b).
5. Sponsoring the PsycINFO database (see Chapter 13).

Deficits in Professional Organizations' Resources

While these resources offered by professional organizations are certainly valuable, they also may be insufficient. As EBP gains momentum, more clinicians will want to learn how to incorporate research into their practice, and their professional organizations will need to find additional ways to support clinicians through this culture shift. Rather than providing access to journal articles and the occasional workshop or online class, professional organizations of the future might need to devote conferences to addressing research-informed practice and offer a greater number of classes geared specifically toward helping clinicians adopt EBP.

When the McMaster's group initially summarized EBP principles, the American Medical Association published a series of articles in the *Journal of the American Medical Association* that described necessary skills and knowledge for EBP (Guyatt & Rennie, 1993). Eventually, these teaching articles were published as a manual and formed into a multitude of presentations at conferences in order to introduce EBP skills to clinicians (Guyatt, Rennie, Meade, & Cook, 2008). Since then, mental health organizations have followed the lead of medical groups.

However, many challenges to EBP in mental health still exist. Professional organizations recognize that some of the most popular models and theories used by their members have little empirical support. In addition, unlike medicine, therapy is often an ongoing process instead of a linear cause-and-effect event. Therapists may be reluctant for their organizations to try to mirror medical groups because they fear that the unique qualities of their paradigm will be lost. In addition, professional organizations, as advocates for their members, struggle with obtaining payment for their members as funders increasingly demand proof of the effectiveness of their treatment approaches. Professional organizations have limited resources and must depend on others to provide funding for research to develop and evaluate evidence-based treatments. Finally, there is an inherent competition among these organizations as resources and funding become scarce. As a result, most professional organizations work in isolation with limited resources instead of combining efforts.

It might be beneficial for professional organizations to share resources in order to identify the most-effective means of helping therapists implement EBP. This would aid professional organizations in choosing where to put their limited resources. For example, spending money on experiential workshops might be weighed against spending money on computer-assisted learning tools. As mentioned previously, some medical associations require reviewers and authors to provide a "grade" for the quality of evidence they offer to support their recommendations. These newly created extra steps for publication require both additional time and expense. Still, most mental health journals will have to update their regulations if they are going to stay abreast of EBP standards.

THE INFLUENCE OF THE INTERNET ON CLINICIANS AND CONSUMERS

As technology advances, information about EBP is becoming more accessible to clinicians through the Internet. As with any other topic, there are good EBP Internet resources, which experts have created or reviewed, as well as some misleading sources of information. Some resources are created for professionals (e.g., *www.essentialevidenceplus. com*; *www.ebbp.org*) while others are created for consumers (e.g., *www. webmd.com*; *www.mayoclinic.com*). However, many recent resources are available to both consumers/patients and health care providers (e.g., *www.supersmarthealth.com*; *www.uptodate.com*). Increasingly, the boundary between consumer and professional information may be blurred. For example, the United States government frequently offers evidence-based information and resources simultaneously to both clients and providers.

In addition to assisting professionals, the Internet will also play a vital role in helping clients learn about evidence-based treatments. A new generation has grown up with the Internet, which individuals routinely use to gather information—including information about mental health care. As resources like SuperSmartHealth and UpToDate become more widespread, consumers will have increased access to research-based knowledge online. Just as patients might look up weight-loss strategies or diabetes treatments online, consumers might begin to do the same for couple therapy, family therapy, or treatment of various psychiatric disorders.

Current research on medical decision making has revealed that while patients still value the opinion of their health care provider over information that they find on the Internet, some patients do consider the Internet to be very important in making medical decisions with their physicians (Couper et al., 2010). Mathieu (2010) points out that there are many people who do not go to the doctor when they experience symptoms, and hypothesizes that this might be because they are using the Internet to make medical decisions on their own. In such instances, the Internet is playing a crucial role in how consumers interact with the health care system.

Similar issues may occur with behavioral and mental health issues. For example, rather than seeing a clinician regarding sexual difficulties, individuals might conduct a Google search on their symptoms, diagnose themselves with a sexual dysfunction (or determine on their own that they are fine), and then choose how to proceed. This might mean seeing a clinician, or it might mean conducting further online searches for do-it-yourself treatments.

In fact, within some health care organizations, systems are being created with the assumption that patients will (somewhat) manage their own health through advanced information and communication technologies. Therefore, the role of seeking information online will likely grow.

For example, a key goal of the patient-centered medical home (PCMH) is to promote the use of technology to enhance physician–patient communication and to encourage patients to assume greater responsibility for their health care needs beyond scheduling an appointment with their physician (Edwards et al., in press).

Given that the Internet is important for a large number of people (whether they actually go to the doctor or not), it is important that the future of EBP includes a greater number of high-quality resources for consumers who are using the Internet. Perhaps the future limitations determining access to information will depend more upon the client's education level and other measures of socioeconomic status. Access to computers in the home, familiarity with websites, and adequate knowledge to interpret findings all depend on education level and financial resources. Still, clients will increasingly type in keywords to search engines before they ever cross the threshold of the therapist's office.

As consumers have greater access to evidence-based knowledge, their expectations of clinicians may change. More clients might ask for empirical support when therapists explain treatment options. If clients' demand for EBP increases, therapists will need to be prepared to meet the requirement.

CONCLUSION

Although not all clinicians choose to incorporate EBP into their work, the EBP movement is gaining momentum and support across disciplines. As the demand for EBP increases, educators, professional organizations, Internet resources, the managed care system, and consumers will all shape the way that clinicians find, evaluate, and apply evidence-based knowledge. We hope that you will consider using research to inform your clinical practice. If you do, remember that there are resources available to help you with this endeavor.

We also would like to leave you with one word of caution: Research evidence is ever-changing and should not be considered a be-all, end-all source of information. Scientists are human, and so research is imperfect. Not all research evidence is good. We hope that as you begin to integrate research into your clinical practice, you will remember this and exercise caution: Just because it was published does not mean it is reliable, valid, or ethical. Using this text as well as other resources, learn to evaluate the merits of research studies for yourself so that you can avoid costly mistakes.

Cautionary tales aside, research is a truly invaluable resource for clinicians. By reviewing the research literature, clinicians can learn about the effectiveness of certain treatments, with which people those treatments are most effective, therapist and client characteristics that shape client outcomes, and common obstacles to look out for in certain cases. At its best, research evidence allows us to reveal lasting truths about nature. After all, it was evidence that allowed us to understand our universe. We believe that combining evidence with the knowledge you have gained from your clinical experience and your understanding of the nuances of your client's lives will make your clinical practice more rewarding for you as well as your clients.

Evidence-Based Practice Pocket Guide (the Five A's)

ASK (STEP 1)

Convert the need for information into an answerable question (Chapter 13).

1. Define the purpose of the search. The five types of questions by Gibbs (2003) can help define the purpose: effectiveness, prevention, risk/prognosis, assessment, and description. You can further define questions using W words (*who, what, where, when, why*) or PICO (**P**atient group or population, **I**ntervention, **C**omparison group, **O**utcome measures).
2. Frame the question using appropriate keywords. Keywords can be found in reference titles and database thesauruses.

ACQUIRE (STEP 2)

Locate the best evidence to answer your questions (Chapter 13).

1. Decide on whether to look for primary (original research) or secondary sources (summaries or reviews of original research).
2. Decide which database(s) you want to search.
3. If necessary, expand your search by (a) looking in other databases, (b) expanding possible keywords, (c) using the references in articles you have found to identify other research, or (d) identifying research that cites articles you have already found.
4. If necessary, narrow the search by (a) limiting the search using various criteria (date of publication, methodology, type of publication, etc.), or (b) developing more specific questions (e.g., ODD *and* ADHD, rather than each separately).

245

APPRAISE (STEP 3)

The following criteria can be used to critically evaluate research studies (Chapters 2–11, 14):

1. Evaluate the study for internal validity concerns.
2. Evaluate the study for external validity concerns.
3. Evaluate the study for measurement concerns.
4. Evaluate the analysis procedures used in the study (statistics, qualitative).
5. Identify other potential concerns (e.g., ethics).

   Note: See Appendix III for more detailed questions for evaluating research studies.

APPLY (STEP 4)

The following questions should be considered when integrating research with clinical expertise, patient preferences, and clinical context (Chapters 15–17):

1. How does my client compare to the samples upon which the studies were conducted (Chapter 15)?
2. How will I know if the treatment will work in the real world (Chapter 15)?
3. Are there multiple problems that need to be addressed within an individual or family? If so, how do you combine different evidence-based treatments (Chapter 15)?
4. How do I learn about the evidence-based treatments I want to use (Chapters 15–16)?
5. How faithful must I be in implementing the evidence-based treatment, or can I modify it based on my client or clinical style (Chapter 15)?
6. How do I involve the client in making decisions about using evidence-based treatments (e.g., informed consent, shared decision making) (Chapters 15 and 17)?

ANALYZE AND ADJUST (STEP 5)

Evaluate your therapy to measure how effective your treatment is (Chapter 18).

1. Can use instruments like the Session Rating Scale, the STIC, Couple Therapy Alliance Scale, Family Therapy Alliance Scale, and others to evaluate the therapy process (e.g., therapeutic alliance).
2. Can use instruments like the Outcome Rating Scale, the STIC, OQ-45, and others to evaluate progress in therapy.

Guide to Evaluating
Research Studies

GENERAL CONSIDERATIONS
FOR EVALUATING RESEARCH STUDIES

Literature Review

1. Does the author make a convincing argument as to the need for the study?
2. Are the research questions and purpose of the study clearly stated?
3. Does the literature review cover all the salient research?
4. Does the literature review include the most recent available research?
5. Does the author provide a critique of the research, or is it simply described?

Methods

1. Is the research design clearly described, including the procedures followed?
2. What implications does the design have for internal validity?
3. Are there any ethical implications for how the study was done (e.g., deception)?
4. Does the study clearly describe the sampling procedures used?
5. How do the sampling procedures (e.g., probability, nonprobability sampling) impact external validity?
6. Do inclusion or exclusion criteria impact the external validity of the findings?
7. Are the sample demographics adequately described?
8. Are there concerns about the sample size?

9. Do attrition or response rates impact the study?
10. Does the study adequately describe the instruments or measures used in the study?
11. Do the instruments or measures have good reliability and validity?
12. Are there other concerns about the instrument or measures used in terms of sensitivity or reactivity?
13. Are the types of analyses clearly and adequately described?
14. Do the types of statistical analyses seem appropriate?
15. For statistical analyses, does the research specify how missing data were handled?
16. For statistical analyses, does the research make explicit if underlying assumptions were examined (e.g., normality, outliers)?

Results and Discussion

1. Does the author draw reasonable conclusions based on the research results?
2. Are the potential limitations of the research adequately addressed?
3. Are potential directions for future research suggested?
4. Does the researcher discuss the clinical significance of the research (not just statistical significance)?
5. Does the researcher address potential clinical or policy implications from the research?

QUESTIONS FOR EVALUATING SPECIFIC DESIGNS

Experimental or Outcome Research (Chapters 3 and 7)

1. Did the experimental design include a comparison group (e.g., control, treatment as usual)?
2. Did the experimental design use randomization of subjects?
3. Did the research do any testing to confirm equivalence of groups?
4. Was the experiment designed to rule out placebo effects?
5. Was the experiment designed to rule out attention effects?
6. To what extent was mortality (especially selective mortality) a potential issue?
7. Are there any other threats to internal validity for an RCT (e.g., compensatory rivalry, diffusion)?
8. Did the research use reliable and valid measures for assessing outcomes?
9. Did the researcher use self-report and/or behavioral measures of outcome?

10. Did the study measure changes in the presenting problem and/or changes in the family dynamics?
11. Did the research measure whether therapists delivered the treatments as intended?
12. To what extent do inclusion or exclusion criteria impact the ability to generalize the findings?
13. Are there aspects of the treatment that would be difficult to implement in the real world?

Survey Research (Chapter 5)

1. Is the purpose of the study clearly stated?
2. Does the researcher adequately describe the sampling approach (e.g., probability, nonprobability) used in the study?
3. What are the implications of the sampling method on external validity?
4. How does the response rate impact external validity?
5. Does the researcher acknowledge limits to external validity based on the sampling procedures used?
6. Did the researcher provide sufficient information about the survey, including the reliability and validity of any established measures incorporated into the survey?
7. If the survey is available, consider the following questions:
   a. Are there any concerns with the wording of questions (e.g., confusing, double-barreled, leading)?
   b. Are there any concerns with the response categories (e.g., number of choices, mutually exclusive, exhaustive)?
   c. Are there any concerns with the ordering of questions?
   d. For questionnaires, are there any concerns with formatting?
8. Was the survey piloted to identify potential problems with the survey?
9. For interviews, is there evidence that the interviewers were properly trained?
10. Does the researcher acknowledge limits to internal validity if the data is correlational?

Qualitative Research (Chapter 6)

1. Is the purpose of the study clearly defined?
2. Are the guiding research questions articulated?
3. For ethnographies, is the setting clearly described? How will the selection of the setting impact the study findings?

4. Is the sampling approach (e.g., selection criteria) clearly described?
5. How will the sampling method impact the study findings?
6. Is the sample adequately described?
7. Does the study clearly define the researcher's role?
8. Was the background, theoretical orientation, and potential biases of the researcher described?
9. Were the types of data clearly explained, including how the data were collected?
10. Were enough data collected to reach saturation?
11. Did the study clearly describe how the data were analyzed (e.g., constant comparative analysis)?
12. Did the researcher state what methods were used to ensure the trustworthiness of the data (e.g., triangulation, member checking)?
13. Did the researcher provide adequate quotes or narratives (e.g., "rich-thick descriptions") to support the findings?

Meta-Analysis (Chapter 7)

1. Did the researcher clearly state what types of studies were included (e.g., published, unpublished, type of experimental design)?
2. How does the criteria impact the findings from the study?
3. Is there a potential for a publication bias if only published studies were included?
4. Was the researcher exhaustive in locating potential studies based on the databases and keywords used in the search?
5. Did the researcher make explicit how the meta-analysis was conducted (e.g., how the effect size was calculated)?
6. Did the researcher rate aspects of the studies (e.g., methodological strength, type of outcome measures) to see if they were related to the effect size?
7. Was an influence analysis conducted?
8. What is the clinical significance of the findings based on the reported effect size?

Reversal (ABA and ABAB) and Multiple-Baseline Designs (Chapter 7)

1. Is the treatment clearly described?
2. Is there evidence that the treatment was delivered as expected?
3. For reversal designs, did the researcher use an ABA design, or the stronger ABAB design?

4. Was the change in measured behavior pronounced when the treatment was introduced or withdrawn?

5. How many subjects were in the study, and how does it impact the confidence in internal validity? This will be especially important for multiple-baseline designs.

6. Did the rescarcher provide a clear description of the subjects so you can evaluate external validity when applying the findings to others?

Content Analysis (Chapter 7)

1. Did the researcher clearly describe the coding systems?

2. Do the coding systems have good interrater reliability?

3. Does the researcher provide a good rationale regarding which materials (e.g., journals) were included for analysis? Do you have any concerns about how representative the materials are?

4. If the study sampled a portion of the eligible materials, was the sampling conducted in an appropriate fashion?

5. Did the researcher draw appropriate conclusions from the content analysis, particularly in relationship to external validity?

Observational Research (Chapter 7)

1. Does the researcher adequately describe the coding system?

2. Are the categories for the coding system clearly defined, exhaustive, and mutually exclusive (if applicable)?

3. Does the coding system have good interrater reliability?

4. Is there evidence for the validity of the coding system?

5. Does the study describe any steps that the researcher used to ensure the coders properly used the coding system?

6. Are there issues regarding external validity based on the type of sample used?

7. Are there issues regarding internal validity based on the type of design (e.g., experimental, nonexperimental) or type of data (e.g., correlational)?

Cross-Sectional and Longitudinal Research (Chapter 7)

1. For cross-sectional research, what are possible cohort effects? Does the researcher do an adequate job of addressing this issue?

2. For longitudinal research, how many participants have been lost over time? Are the individuals who have dropped out over time different in a significant way from those who remain?

QUESTIONS FOR EVALUATING REVIEWS

1. Is the purpose of the review clearly stated?
2. Does the review explicitly state what steps were taken to locate the research (e.g., databases searched, keywords)?
3. Does the search appear to be exhaustive based on steps described above?
4. Does the review clearly articulate the criteria used to determine if a study was to be included or excluded in the review?
5. Were multiple reviewers used? Are there any concerns about the review process (e.g., biases)?
6. Does the review describe the studies in the review in sufficient detail (e.g., sample size, type of experimental design)?
7. Does the review evaluate the rigor or quality of the studies included?
8. Do the conclusions make sense based on the review of the findings across studies?
9. Does the review offer a perspective on the strength of evidence for the conclusions?
10. Does the review note possible limitations and implications for future research?

Evidenced–Based
Practice Resources

EVIDENCE-BASED PRACTICE TRAINING MODULES

If you are interested in online tutorials for evidence-based practice, you might explore the Evidence-Based Behavioral Practice website (*www.ebbp.org/training. html*) or the Columbia University School of Social Work website (*www.columbia. edu/cu/musher/Website/Website/EBP_OnlineTraining.htm*). In addition, the University of Alberta has an Evidence-Based Medicine Toolkit with valuable resources (*www.ebm.med.ualberta.ca*).

RESOURCES AND TUTORIALS
FOR SEARCHING DATABASES

In Chapter 13, we discussed searching databases for research. Table 13.1 summarizes several databases with which you will want to be familiar. There are also online resources for learning how to use some of the more important databases like PsycINFO (*www.apa.org/pubs/databases/training/index.aspx*) and PubMed (*www.nlm.nih.gov/bsd/disted/pubmed.html*). In addition, the Evidence-Based Behavioral Practice website offers videos on searching the following databases:

Cochrane Library
www.ebbp.org/course_outlines/searching_for_evidence/video/EBBP-Cochrane/EBBP-Cochrane.htm

PsycINFO
www.ebbp.org/course_outlines/searching_for_evidence/video/EBBP-PsycInfo/EBBP-PsycInfo.htm

PubMed, Part 1
*www.ebbp.org/course_outlines/searching_for_evidence/video/EBBP-PubMed_
part1/EBBP-PubMed_part1.htm*

PubMed, Part 2
*www.ebbp.org/course_outlines/searching_for_evidence/video/EBBP-PubMed_
part2/EBBP-PubMed_part2.htm*

CLINICAL BOOKS FOR LEARNING
EVIDENCE-BASED TREATMENTS

In Chapter 17, we discussed various couple- and family-based treatments with
empirical support that you may want to use when working with commonly
encountered family and couple problems. If you are interested in exploring any
of these approaches further, you may want to consult the following books:

- **Functional Family Therapy**—Alexander, J. F., Waldron, H. B., Robbins, M. S., & Neeb, A. A. (2013). *Functional family therapy for adolescent behavior problems.* Washington, DC: American Psychological
  Association; or Sexton, T. L. (2011). *Functional family therapy in clinical
  practice: An evidence-based treatment model for working with troubled adolescents.* New York: Routledge.
- **Brief Strategic Family Therapy**—A free manual entitled *Brief Strategic Family Therapy for Adolescent Drug Abuse* can be found at *http://
  ctndisseminationlibrary.org/display/32.htm.*
- **Multisystemic Therapy**—Henggeler, W., Schoenwald, S. K., Borduin,
  C. M., Rowland, M. D., & Cunningham, P. B. (2009). *Multisystemic
  therapy for antisocial behavior in children and adolescents* (2nd ed.). New
  York: Guilford Press.
- **Multidimensional Family Therapy**—**Multidimensional Family
  Therapy for Adolescent Cannabis Users** (2002) is available for free
  from SAMHSA at *shttp://store.samhsa.gov/product/Multidimensional-
  Family-Therapy-for-Adolescent-Cannabis-Users/BKD388.*
- **Parent Management Training**—Kazdin, A. E. (2005). *Parent manage-
  ment training: Treatment for oppositional, aggressive, and antisocial behav-
  ior in children and adolescents.* New York: Oxford University Press.
- **Parent-Child Interaction Therapy**—McNeil, C. B., & Hembree-Kigin,
  T. L. (2011). *Parent–child interaction therapy* (2nd ed.). New York: Springer.
- **Maudsley Approach for Eating Disorders**—Treasure, J., Schmidt, U.,
  & Macdonald, P. (Eds.). (2009). *The clinician's guide to collaborative car-
  ing in eating disorders: The new Maudsley method.* New York: Routledge.
- **Family Psychoeducation for Severe Mental Illness**—McFarlane, W.

R. (2002). *Multifamily groups in the treatment of severe psychiatric disorders.* New York: Guilford Press.

- **Behavioral Couples Therapy for Substance Abuse**—O'Farrell, T. J., & Fals-Stewart, W. (2006). *Behavioral couples therapy for alcoholism and drug abuse.* New York: Guilford Press.
- **Gottman Method Couple Approach**—Gottman, J. M. (1999). *The marriage clinic: A scientifically based marital therapy.* New York: Norton.
- **Emotionally Focused Therapy**—Johnson, S. M. (2004). *The practice of emotionally focused couple therapy: Creating connection* (2nd ed.). New York: Brunner-Routledge.
- **Integrative Behavioral Couple Therapy**—Jacobson, N. S., & Christensen, A. (1998). *Acceptance and change in couple therapy: A therapist's guide to transforming relationships.* New York: Norton.
- **Cognitive Behavioral Couple Therapy**—Epstein, N., & Baucom, D. H. (2002). *Enhanced cognitive-behavioral couple therapy for couples: A contextual approach.* Washington, DC: American Psychological Association.
- **Infidelity or Affairs**—Baucom, D. H., Snyder, D. K., & Gordon, K. C. (2009). *Helping couples get past the affair: A clinician's guide.* New York: Guilford Press.

INSTRUMENTS FOR MEASURING
THERAPY PROCESS AND OUTCOMES

In Chapter 18, we discussed various measures for evaluating therapy process and outcome, which are listed below:

Measures for Therapeutic Alliance

- Session Rating Scale (SRS)
- Working Alliance Inventory (WAI)
- Couple Therapy Alliance Scale (CTAS) and Family Therapy Alliance Scale (FTAS)
- Vanderbilt Therapeutic Alliance Scale (VTAS)
- System for Observing Family Therapy Alliances (SOFTA)
- Intersession STIC

Measures for Therapeutic Outcome

- Outcome Questionnaire–45 (OQ-45) and Youth Outcome Questionnaire (Y-OQ)
- Outcome Rating Scale (ORS)
- Systemic Inventory of Change (STIC)

GOVERNMENT AGENCIES AND INITIATIVES THAT SUPPORT EVIDENCE-BASED PRACTICE IN HEALTH CARE

In Chapter 19, we discussed the importance of different government agencies or initiatives in promoting EBP in health care. For more information about these agencies, you can visit the following websites:

- Agency for Healthcare Research and Quality (AHRQ; *www.ahrq.gov*)
- United States Preventive Services Task Force (USPSTF; *www.ahrq.gov/ clinic/uspstfix.htm*)
- Translating Research Into Practice (TRIP-II; *www.ahrq.gov/research/ trip2fac.htm*)

OTHER RESOURCES

Throughout the book we have mentioned organizations or groups that you may want to explore further to learn more about their work related to EBP. These include the following:

- The American Academy of Child and Adolescent Psychiatry has a website (*www.aacap.org/AACAP/Resources_for_Primary_Care/Practice_ Parameters_and_Resource_Centers/Practice_Parameters.aspx*) that provides recommendations for treating and assessing children and adolescents with psychiatric disorders.
- The American Psychiatric Association has a website (*www.psych.org/ practice/clinical-practice-guidelines*) that provides clinical practice guidelines for treating common psychiatric illnesses among adults.
- The American Psychological Association, Division 12, has a website (*www.div12.org/PsychologicalTreatments*) that lists research-supported treatments for various adult psychological disorders. The site indicates how strong the evidence is for each treatment (e.g., strong support, modest support), as well as a brief description of it.
- The American Psychological Association, Division 53, has a website (*http://effectivechildtherapy.com*) that lists research-supported treatments for various psychological disorders specific to children and adolescents. The site indicates how strong the evidence is for each listed treatment (e.g., well established, probably efficacious, possibly efficacious), as well as a brief description of many of the treatments.
- CONSORT (*www.consort-statement.org*) has developed guidelines or standards for reporting randomized controlled trials (RCTs).
- The GRADE working group (*www.gradeworkinggroup.org*) has developed a system for grading the quality of evidence for treatment recommendations.

Glossary

ABA design—A research design in which the researcher evaluates the impact of administering and withdrawing the treatment to see if the treatment had an effect. The researcher first establishes a baseline (A) before administering the treatment. The treatment (B) is then administered to determine if it has a positive effect. The treatment is then withdrawn (A) to see if the problem returns to baseline.

ABAB design—A research design that adds an additional step to the ABA design (see above) whereby the researcher administers the treatment again (B) and measures its impact. If reintroducing the treatment creates another positive change, then the researcher has even more confidence that the effect is due to treatment and not some other factor.

Acquire—The second step of the evidence-based process (five A's) where one attempts to locate research literature to answer your question.

Aggregate data—A type of data reporting that combines individual responses and only reports summary statistics such as percentages, averages, or median scores. Aggregating the data makes it impossible to know how any one individual responded, thus protecting each person's privacy.

Alpha—*See* level of significance.

Alternative hypothesis—This hypothesis states that the observed result in a sample reflects what is real in the population, and is not an artifact of sampling error.

Analytical framework—Patterns, themes, typologies, or theories that are inductively derived through qualitative research.

Analyze and adjust—The fifth step of the evidence-based process (the five A's) where one evaluates the effectiveness and efficiency of the chosen treatment.

ANCOVA (analysis of covariance)—A statistical analysis that is similar to ANOVA, except it allows for one of the independent variables to be continuous rather than categorical.

Anonymity—A research design in which the researcher does not know the research participants' identities, which provides greater protection than confidentiality.

ANOVA (analysis of variance)—An inferential statistical test that can be used to measure if the mean scores are different between two or more groups.

Apply—The fourth step of the evidence-based process (the five A's) where one determines how to use the research clinically, taking into account a number of factors such as clinical expertise, client preferences, and context.

Appraise—The third step of the evidence-based process (the five A's) where one evaluates the quality of the research evidence.

Ask—The initial step of the evidence-based process (the five A's) where one creates a question that can be answered by the research literature.

Autoethnography—A type of qualitative research where the goal is to provide a reflexive account of the researcher's life and how it relates to his or her culture.

Canonical correlation—A statistical analysis in which multiple independent variables are used to predict multiple dependent variables.

Ceiling effects—This occurs when scores from a multi-item scale cluster on the high end, thereby reducing sensitivity.

Chi-square—A bivariate statistical test that is used to determine if there is a relationship between two categorical variables.

Clinical significance—A term that relates to whether the results of a study have practical significance and are meaningful regarding real-life applications.

Closed-ended questions—Questions that offer the respondent choices from which to select.

Coding system—A system with predetermined categories developed by the researcher for recording data.

Cohort effects—The effects of being born at a similar time in history, exposed to the same events in society, and influenced by the same demographic trends, and thus having similar experiences that differentiate the group from other groups. This can be a threat to interval validity in cross-sectional research because it is possible that differences found between the groups could be due to each group (cohort) having a different history.

Concurrent validity—A type of measurement validity that is established by correlating the new instrument with a criterion variable known concurrently or at the same time (rather than the future).

Confidence interval—The range in which a population value is expected to fall within based on the sample characteristics (e.g., sample size, standard deviation), assuming a certain confidence level (typically 95%). The confidence interval is also called the margin of error.

Confidentiality—A legal and ethical concept in research relating to restrictions on disclosure of the identities of participants to anyone outside the study.

Constant comparative method—A process for analyzing qualitative data in which the researcher continually sorts and categorizes new observations, which over time results in an emerging analytical framework for understanding the phenomenon.

Construct—A label used to represent a phenomenon that is not directly observable. Constructs are abstract concepts (e.g., love, marital satisfaction) that cannot be directly measured, unlike physical properties (e.g., weight, length).

Construct validity—This type of measurement validity is demonstrated by showing that the instrument relates to other constructs as theoretically expected.

Content analysis—A method of studying the content of some form of recorded media or communication, such as TV shows, movies, speeches, or publications. In family therapy, content analysis often examines the content of journal articles to see what trends are evident in the field.

Content validity—A type of measurement validity that evaluates if the instrument includes all the important aspects of the construct.

Convenience sampling—A nonprobability sampling method in which the researcher uses a sample that is easily available. This type of sampling is also referred to as *availability sampling, accidental sampling, haphazard sampling,* or *opportunity sampling.*

Convergent validity—This type of measurement validity is demonstrated by showing that the instrument strongly correlates with another way of measuring the same construct.

Conversation analysis—A qualitative design in which a conversation or dialogue between individuals is recorded and analyzed to gain insight into the dynamics of the relationship.

Criterion validity—This type of measurement validity is demonstrated by showing that the new instrument relates to another criterion or indicator in an anticipated manner.

Cross-sectional research—A research design in which individuals (or relationships) of different ages are studied at the same time to see how they are similar and different. Cross-sectional research attempts to study how things change over time.

Deductive—A type of reasoning that moves from general to specific. For example, the researcher takes a theory (general) and derives or deduces specific hypotheses from it. Studies are then designed to generate data to test these hypotheses.

Demand characteristics—A form of reactivity that occurs when individuals provide answers that they believe the researcher desires, perhaps to please the researcher or to avoid being judged.

Dependent variable—The variable that is changed by its relationship to other variables (i.e., independent variables). In experimental research, this is the outcome variable.

Discriminant function analysis (DFA)—A multivariate analysis that can be used if the dependent variable is categorical and all of the independent variables are continuous.

Discriminant validity—This type of measurement validity is demonstrated by confirming that the instrument does not strongly correlate with instruments that measure other constructs.

Double-barreled questions—Questions that inquire about more than one thing at a time. Double-barreled questions often include the words *and* or *or* in the questions.

Effect size—A statistic used in meta-analysis that converts data in individual studies into a standardized score. This allows one to compare or compile results across studies.

Effectiveness research or studies—Experimental research studies that are done in real-world clinical settings.

Efficacy research or studies—Experimental studies that are more carefully controlled, such as random control trials. Efficacy studies are prioritized above effectiveness studies when determining evidence-based practices (EBP) status because they are best able to demonstrate that a treatment alone caused change in outcome.

Ethnography—The study of cultures or social groups using a qualitative research design where the researcher immerses him or herself in the culture or setting being studied. Insights about the social group are obtained through observation, interviews, or analyzing documents and other cultural artifacts (e.g., newspapers, letters).

Evidence-based practice (EBP)—The integration of research evidence, clinical expertise, and client values to inform clinical decision making.

Exhaustive—A term used to describe when the responses available to answer a question include all of the possible answers to that question.

External validity—A concept that refers to how far conclusions from a study can be generalized to a larger population. External validity is largely determined by how representative the sample is relative to the people or phenomenon to which the researcher wants to generalize.

Face validity—A type of measurement validity that simply requires that one look at the instrument to judge if it appears to be valid.

Factor analysis—A statistical procedure that correlates each item in a multi-item scale with every other item and then groups correlated items into factors. Using factor analysis, researchers can explore or confirm (see *factorial validity*) what dimensions exist, as well as which items relate to each dimension.

Factorial designs—An experimental design with one outcome variable and two or more independent variables (factors). Factorial designs can test whether each factor has an independent effect (i.e., main effect) or if there is an interaction effect between the factors.

Factorial validity—This type of measurement validity is demonstrated by running a factor analysis to confirm the instrument behaves theoretically as expected with regards to its internal structure or dimensions.

Floor effects—Occurs when scores of a multi-item scale cluster on the low end, thereby reducing sensitivity.

Focus groups—A type of qualitative research where the researcher gathers individuals together to discuss a particular topic. These groups are typically recorded, transcribed, and the content is then analyzed using qualitative methods.

Frequency distribution—A summary of how often different scores occur for a variable within a sample. Frequency distributions can be displayed in tables or histograms (bar graphs).

Funneling—A technique used in creating surveys in which survey questions progress from general to specific in nature.

Grounded theory—A theory that has been developed inductively from qualitative data.

h-index—A measure of an impact for author or journal. The h-index represents the h-number of articles that have been cited at least h times by an author or a journal.

Hierarchical—An approach in which the independent variables enter the multivariate analysis (e.g., multiple regression) in sets according to the researcher's preferences. The order is usually determined by theory.

History—External events that happen during an experiment that can influence the results and thus be a threat to internal validity.

Impact factor—A measure of impact for a journal that is published in the *Journal Citation Reports*. The impact factor is the number of citations found in a particular year for all eligible articles published in the 2 preceding years in a journal, and then dividing this number by the number of eligible articles.

In-depth interviews—A common type of qualitative research in which participants are asked to share their experience regarding a particular topic.

Independent variable—In correlational research, this is the variable that is used to predict another variable in a study. In experimental research, the independent variable is the variable (e.g., treatment) that is manipulated or changed by the researcher.

Inductive—A type of reasoning that derives generalities from specifics (e.g., derive patterns, themes, or theory from specific data).

Inferential statistics—Various statistical analyses that calculate the probability that a sample result is due to sampling error. Inferential statistics are used to help the researcher decide if the sample results are likely due to sampling error or reflect something real in the population.

Influence analysis—A statistical method that identifies which studies in a meta-analysis have the most impact on the overall effect size.

Informed consent—A legal and ethical concept in research and therapy in which individuals should be told important information prior to participation, such as the purpose, potential benefits or risks from participating, and how their privacy/confidentiality will be protected. Based on this information, individuals can then decide whether it is appropriate for them to participate.

Instrument decay—A potential threat to internal validity that occurs when the way the outcome variable is measured changes over time.

Internal reliability—A type of reliability that assesses if all the items in an instrument are consistent in measuring the same construct.

Internal validity—A concept that is concerned with accurately identifying cause and effect relationships between variables. Internal validity involves carefully ruling out competing explanations for why something happens.

Interrater reliability—A type of reliability that assesses the consistency across raters in how they code or categorize behaviors.

Interval—A level of measurement in which the distance (interval) between values is equal, but there is no absolute zero on the scale.

Judgment sampling—*See* Purposive sampling.

Leading questions—Questions that encourage respondents to answer in a particular way, thereby biasing the results.

Learning—A form of reactivity that occurs when the research participant gains knowledge or skills through being measured. This is most likely to occur if an instrument is administered more than once, resulting in improved performance on subsequent administrations through learning new information or repetitive practice.

Level of Significance—This refers to how small the *p*-value is required to be in order to reject the null hypothesis and assume the alternative hypothesis is true. The most common convention is to use .05 or .01 as the level of significance. The level of significance is also called the alpha.

Loading—A technique used when asking questions to address the underreporting of negative behaviors. Loading prefaces the question with a statement that gives the respondent permission for engaging in a socially undesirable behavior.

Logistic regression—A multivariate statistical analysis that can be used if the dependent variable is categorical and the independent variables are either continuous or categorical.

Longitudinal research—A research design in which data is collected from one set of individuals (or relationships) and then the same set of individuals is measured after a certain length of time to see how they have changed.

MANOVA (multivariate analysis of variance)—A multivariate statistical analysis that examines the relationship between a single independent variable that is categorical and multiple dependent variables. MANOVA allows the researcher to test if the mean scores for multiple dependent variables are different for individuals who belong to different groups (independent variable).

Manualized treatments—Treatments where the researcher describes in detail, using a manual, the protocol for delivering the treatment.

Margin of error—*See* Confidence interval.

Maturation—A potential threat to internal validity that can arise due to the fact that people inevitably change over time.

Mean—The arithmetic average of the scores. The mean is calculated by finding the sum of all the scores, then dividing the sum by the number of scores.

Measure of central tendency—A descriptive statistic that attempts to capture the value upon which most of the scores are centered. Mean, median, and mode are all measures of central tendency.

Median—The middle value if the scores are arranged from lowest to highest. (It is the mean of the two middle scores if there is an even number of data points.)

Member checking—A method of ensuring the trustworthiness of qualitative research findings in which the researcher's findings are shared with the research participants prior to publication to confirm that they accurately reflected their experiences.

Memory recall—The ability to accurately remember events or information from the past.

Meta-analysis—A statistical method that is used to combine and contrast results across multiple studies in a particular area. Meta-analysis calculates and then compiles effect size across individual studies.

Micro-theories—Theories that can guide therapists in their moment-to-moment decisions in therapy. Process research can aid in the development of micro-theories.

Mixed methods research—Research that combines both quantitative and qualitative approaches.

Mode—The most frequently occurring score. There can be more than one mode.

Mortality—A potential threat to internal validity that occurs when individuals drop out of a study due to death or some other reason.

Multiple-baseline design—A research design in which the researcher first measures a baseline for each individual in the study. Next, the treatment is staggered across individuals so no one receives the treatment at the same time. If each person improves after receiving the treatment, then the change is likely due to the treatment rather than outside factors that would likely impact study participants simultaneously.

Multiple R—A statistic used in multiple regression that tells us the correlation between the independent variables and the dependent variable. Multiple R can range from 0 (no correlation) to 1 (a perfect correlation).

Multiple regression—A multivariate statistical analysis that allows a researcher to use more than one independent variable to predict a dependent variable.

Multistage cluster sampling—A probability sampling method that can be used when a single list of the entire population does not exist. The researcher first identifies a list of groups or clusters that contain individuals in the population. Then, some of these clusters are randomly selected for further sampling. This process is repeated until the researcher has clusters or subgroups that list the individuals. In the final stage, individuals are randomly selected from these clusters.

Multivariate statistics—Inferential statistics (e.g., multiple regression, logistic regression) that use a combination of three or more independent and dependent variables.

Mutually exclusive—A term used to describe a set of responses to a question in which only one answer can apply to each individual.

Nominal—The lowest level of measurement in which the variables do not have any numeric or quantitative properties and the researcher simply assigns names to the possible choices (e.g., marital status, gender, religious affiliation).

Nonprobability sampling—A type of sampling in which the likelihood or probability of individuals being selected from the general population is unknown. Because not everyone has an equal or known chance of being selected, people in the sample may not be representative of the population, resulting in lower external validity.

Normal distribution—An important type of frequency distribution where the scores fall into a symmetrical, bell-shaped distribution. Many phenomena closely approximate a normal distribution, and it may be assumed that variables will have a normal distribution in many statistical analyses.

Null hypothesis—This hypothesis states that the result observed in a sample does not reflect a real relationship in the population, but is simply an artifact of sampling error.

Observational research—*Also called* Systematic observation. A type of research involving the careful measurement and recording of specific behaviors in a specified setting, typically using some type of coding system.

Open-ended questions—Questions that do not require participants to choose from a predetermined set of possible answers and thus allow the participant to answer in any way that they like (e.g., "How do you feel?").

Operationalize—When operationalizing a construct, the researcher chooses which indicators of the construct they want to measure. Thoughts, feelings, or behaviors are examples of indicators that may be used to operationalize a construct.

Ordinal—A level of measurement that is quantitative in nature and allows one to assign a rank order to values, but does not assume equal distances between those values (e.g., sports polls, Likert scales).

Outcome research—A type of research aimed at determining if a treatment is effective, or how its effectiveness may compare to an alternative treatment. Outcome research is typically done using experimental designs, however, reversal and multiple-baseline designs can also be used.

Outliers—Extreme scores that are sometimes found in a frequency distribution. Outliers can be errors in the data or can reflect a unique situation or distinct phenomenon.

***p*-value**—A statistic that represents the probability that the observed relationship in the sample could be due to sampling error.

P4P—Acronym for "pay-for-performance" programs that offer providers cash incentives for meeting optimum performance levels.

Path analysis—A statistical analysis that can be used to study the interrelationship between multiple variables. The interrelationships (or paths) between variables are analyzed through a combination of multiple regression analyses.

Patient-centered medical home (PCMH)—The concept of a PCMH was created to improve primary care by organizing it around patients' needs. Also, working in teams, coordinating care, and tracking progress over time are all important parts of the PCMH.

Pearson's r correlation—A bivariate statistical analysis that is used to evaluate if a relationship exists between two continuous variables (interval or ratio level of measurement) and the strength of the relationship. It also tells you the direction of the relationship based on whether the correlation coefficient is positive or negative.

Peer debriefing—A method of ensuring the trustworthiness of qualitative research findings in which a professional colleague independently reviews the data and coding to determine if he or she would reach a similar conclusion.

Phenomenology—A type of research that seeks to understand how individuals make meaning out of their personal experience.

PICO—An acronym that stands for (1) Patient group or population, (2) Intervention, (3) Comparison group, and (4) Outcome measures. PICO can be used to help formulate questions.

Piloting—A technique in which the researcher pretests the survey by asking individuals to complete the survey and give feedback on the survey so as to identify potential problems.

Placebo effect—A phenomenon where individuals improve because they expect to benefit from the treatment despite receiving a "fake" treatment (e.g., sugar pill).

Population—The group (usually people) to which the researcher is trying to generalize conclusions.

Post-hoc analysis—A follow-up analysis that is done if a statistically significant result is found after an ANOVA analysis. The post-hoc analysis determines which groups are significantly different from one another.

Practice guidelines—Treatment recommendations and summaries based on evidence-based literature.

Predictive validity—This type of measurement validity is demonstrated by showing that the new measure accurately predicts a criterion variable in the future.

Primary source—The original report of a research study (e.g., journal article, dissertation).

Probability sampling—A type of sampling where everyone in the population has an equal chance or known probability of being selected, resulting in a representative sample.

Process research—A type of research that studies how processes occur in therapy, such as the formation of the therapeutic alliance or how change occurs.

Prolonged engagement—A method of ensuring the trustworthiness of qualitative research findings by requiring the researcher spend sufficient time within a culture or social setting to fully understand it.

Purposive sampling—*Also called* Judgment sampling. A nonprobability sampling method in which the selection of participants is guided by the researcher's judgment as to what type of cases will yield the best information to understand the phenomenon.

Qualitative research—A variety of research designs that offer insight into phenomena that are difficult to quantify numerically. Qualitative research relies on description or words to understand a phenomenon.

Quantitative research—A variety of research designs that use numbers to measure and understand phenomena.

Quasi-experimental design—An experimental design that can be used when it is not possible to randomly assign individuals to groups. In this design, the groups receive both a pretest and posttest. By administering a pretest, the researcher can compare the groups to see if they are equivalent before the experiment begins.

Quota sampling—A nonprobability sampling method that attempts to ensure that certain groups are adequately represented in the sample. First, the population is segmented into mutually exclusive subgroups. Convenience sampling is then used to fill each group.

Randomized controlled trial (RCT)—An experimental study design in which participants are randomly assigned to the treatment and comparison groups (e.g., no treatment control, alternative treatment).

Range—A measure of variability that represents the difference between the highest and lowest values.

Ratio—The highest level of measurement that possesses both equal intervals and an absolute zero.

Reactivity—A process describing how individuals who know that they are being observed may change their behavior. Researchers want to minimize reactivity to get a more accurate picture of how people really are.

Reliability—A concept that refers to whether the instrument gives a consistent answer. A measure is said to have a high reliability if it produces similar results under consistent conditions.

Repeated-measures design—A study design in which subjects are exposed to more than one condition and then differences in their responses are measured. In this design, subjects act as their own comparison group. Also called a within-subjects design.

Research questions—Questions that reflect the purpose of the study or what the researcher hopes to learn. These questions are more global in nature than the specific questions asked in a survey.

Response rate—The number of people who completed a survey divided by the entire number of people who were asked to complete the survey. The response rate is often expressed as a percentage.

Reversal designs—Research designs (ABA, ABAB) in which the researcher evaluates the impact of administering and withdrawing the treatment to see if the treatment had an effect. These designs are often employed when there are a limited number of subjects.

Rich–thick descriptions—Quotes or narrative descriptions that are included in the write-up of a qualitative study to illustrate and provide support for the researcher's conclusions.

Sample—A subset of the larger population from which data is collected for a study.

Sampling error—Error due to chance or random factors that may result in a sample not being 100% representative of the population. This can occur even when probability sampling methods are used.

Sampling frame—A list of the population from which the sample is drawn when using probability sampling.

Saturation—A state that occurs during qualitative research when analysis of new cases does not yield any new insights. Analysis of additional cases simply repeats themes or insights found in earlier cases.

Secondary sources—These are sources (e.g., reviews, practice guidelines) that summarize or synthesize information from primary sources.

Selection bias—A potential threat to internal validity that occurs when the individuals select which treatment they will receive, creating the potential for preexisting differences to exist between the groups. As a result, it becomes difficult to determine if the results are due to preexisting differences between the subjects or due to treatment effects.

Self-report instruments—Instruments that ask individuals to volunteer what they are thinking, feeling, or doing.

Sensitivity—The ability of an instrument to detect differences between individuals when measuring a construct.

Shared decision making—A process where the clinician and the client collaboratively decide what is the best approach to treatment.

Simple random sampling—A probability sampling method in which all individuals in the population are assigned a number, which are then randomly selected to create a sample.

Skewed—An asymmetrical frequency distribution in which there are more scores on one side of the curve.

Snowballing—A sampling method in which individuals who meet criteria for the study are asked to recommend others who may also fit the criteria. These individuals, in turn, may be able to identify others who fit the criteria, creating a snowballing effect.

Social desirability—The most common form of reactivity in which individuals answer questions or behave in a manner that makes them appear good. Social desirability leads individuals to overreport positive behaviors and to underreport negative behaviors so they can be viewed in a favorable manner.

Solomon four-group design—A study design in which both the experimental and comparison groups are conducted with and without pretesting, creating four groups. The two experimental groups or two control groups can be compared with one another to see if pretesting created a difference.

Spurious relationship—A relationship where two variables have no direct causal connection, yet it appears that they do. This can arise if both variables are correlated to a third variable.

Standard—An approach in which the independent variables are entered into the multivariate analysis (e.g., multiple regression) simultaneously.

Standard deviation—A measure of variability that is calculated by taking the square root of the variance. The standard deviation is typically reported rather than the variance because it is in the same units as the mean.

Statistical regression to the mean—A phenomenon that describes how some scores are initially extreme due in part to chance factors and that these scores will usually return to their normal baseline upon retesting.

Statistically significant—A term that is used when the researcher rejects the null hypothesis because the p-value from a statistical analysis is equal to or lower than the level of significance (or alpha).

Stepwise—An approach in which the independent variables enter the multivariate analysis (e.g., multiple regression) one at a time based on their ability to predict the dependent variable. At each step, stepwise selects the most powerful predictor among the available variables, and continues this process until all of the significant predictors have been used.

Stratified sampling—A probability sampling method in which the sampling frame or list is divided into strata or groups along important attributes (e.g., ethnicity/race). Simple random sampling or systematic sampling is then used to fill each group or strata.

Structural equation modeling (SEM)—A statistical analysis that can be used to study the interrelationship between multiple constructs. SEM is similar to path analysis in many regards, but uses multiple measures to operationalize constructs with the aid of factor analysis.

Survey—A study design in which the researcher uses questions to gain access to the private thoughts, emotions, and behaviors of individuals.

Systematic observation—*See* Observational research.

Systematic review—A review of the literature that uses a rigorous approach to select, locate, evaluate, and synthesize research studies to answer specific questions.

Systematic sampling—A probability sampling procedure that creates a sample by starting at a random point in the sampling frame list and then choosing every nth person (e.g. every third person).

***t*-test**—An inferential statistic that is used to evaluate whether the mean scores between two groups are different.

Task analysis—A discovery-oriented approach to studying therapy in which researchers study critical events in therapy and try to uncover patterns that lead to either successful or unsuccessful outcomes.

Test–retest reliability—A type of reliability which measures the consistency of scores over time.

Testing—This refers to any potential threat to internal validity due to reactivity.

Theoretical sampling—A sampling procedure in which the researcher chooses specific cases to help in developing an emerging theory by providing additional insight into the selected phenomenon.

Threats to internal validity—These include any competing explanations for why an effect was found other than the hypothesized causal variable.

Translational research—Research that examines what happens when research findings are moved from the researcher's controlled lab to the real world.

Triangulation—A method of ensuring the trustworthiness of qualitative research findings that requires the researcher to collect information from multiple sources to crosscheck the findings.

Type I error—This occurs when the researcher rejects the null hypothesis (assumes the alternative hypothesis is true), but the null hypothesis is actually true.

Type II error—This occurs when the researcher assumes the null hypothesis is true, but the alternative hypothesis is true.

Validity—The extent to which an instrument measures what it claims to measure.

Variance—A measure of variability that is conceptually analogous to finding the average distance of scores from the mean. However, the distance between each score and the mean is squared before finding the average so that the sum of scores will not be zero.

Within-subjects design—*See* Repeated-measures design.

References

Aarons, G. A., Hulbert, M., & McCue Horwitz, S. (2011). Advancing a conceptual model of evidence-based practice implementation in public service sectors. *Administration and Policy in Mental Health and Mental Health Services Research, 38*(1), 4–23.

Agency for Healthcare Research and Quality. (2001). Translating research into practice (TRIP)–II. Fact sheet (AHRQ Publication No. 01-P017). Retrieved April 19, 2012, from *www.ahrq.gov/research/trip2fac.htm*.

Agency for Healthcare Research and Quality. (2011). Evidence-based practice centers overview. Retrieved April 19, 2012, from *www.ahrq.gov/clinic/epc/APA*.

Agency for Healthcare Research and Quality. (2012). Pay for performance (P4P): AHRQ resources. Retrieved August 5, 2012, from *www.ahrq.gov/professionals/ quality-patient-safety/quality-resources/tools/p4p/p4pguide4.html*.

Allen, K. R., & Piercy, F. P. (2005). Feminist autoethnography. In D. H. Sprenkle & F. P. Piercy (Eds.), *Research methods in family therapy* (2nd ed., pp. 155–169). New York: Guilford Press.

Amato, P. R. (2010). Research on divorce: Continuing trends and new developments. *Journal of Marriage and the Family, 72,* 650–666.

American Association for Marriage and Family Therapy. (2012, July 1). AAMFT *code of ethics.* Retrieved September 4, 2013, from *www.aamft.org/imis15/content/ legal_ethics/code_of_ethics.aspx*.

American Psychiatric Association. (2013). *Diagnostic and statistical manual of mental disorders* (5th ed.). Arlington, VA: Author.

American Psychological Association. (2005). *Policy statement on evidence-based practice in psychology.* Retrieved April 19, 2012, from *www.apa.org/practice/ resources/evidence/evidence-based-statement.pdf*.

American Psychological Association. (2012a). *Evidence-based behavioral practice programs.* Retrieved April 19, 2012, from *www.apa.org/ed/ce/resources/ebbp. aspx*.

American Psychological Association. (2012b). *Education: Evidence-based practice in psychology.* Retrieved April 19, 2012, from *www.apa.org/education/ce/1370028. aspx.*

Arora, N. K., & McHorney, C. A. (2000). Patient preferences for medical decision making: Who really wants to participate? *Medical Care, 38*(3), 335–341.

Babbie, E. (1992). *The practice of social research* (6th ed.). Belmont, CA: Thomson Wadsworth.

Babbie, E. (2007). *The practice of social research* (11th ed.). Belmont, CA: Thomson Wadsworth.

Baker, T. B., McFall, R. M., & Shoham, V. (2008). Current status and future prospects of clinical psychology: Toward a scientifically principled approach to mental and behavioral health care. *Psychological Science in the Public Interest, 9*, 67–103.

Baldwin, S. A., Christian, S., Berkeljon, A., Shadish, W. R., & Bean, R. (2012). The effects of family therapies for adolescent delinquency and substance abuse: A meta-analysis. *Journal of Marital and Family Therapy, 38*, 281–304.

Barnes, F. (1995, July). Can you trust those polls? *Reader's Digest, 146*, 49–54.

Barrett, A. (2008). Evidence-based medicine and shared decision making: The challenge of getting both evidence and preferences into health care. *Patient Education and Counseling, 73*(3), 407–412.

Baucom, D. H., Epstein, N. B., LaTaillade, J. J., & Kirby, J. S. (2008). Cognitive-behavioral couple therapy. In A. S. Gurman (Ed.), *Clinical handbook of couple therapy* (4th ed., pp. 31–72). New York: Guilford Press.

Baucom, K. J. W., Sevier, M., Eldridge, K. A., Doss, B. D., & Christensen, A. (2011). Observed communication in couples two years after integrative and traditional behavioral couple therapy: Outcome and link with 5-year follow-up. *Journal of Consulting and Clinical Psychology, 79*, 565–576.

Bauer, R. M. (2007). Evidence-based practice in psychology: Implications for research and research training. *Journal of Clinical Psychology, 73*(7), 685–694.

Beach, R. H., & Whisman, M. A. (2012). Affective disorders. *Journal of Marital and Family Therapy, 38*, 201–219.

Beidas, R. S., & Kendall, P. C. (2010). Training therapists in evidence-based practice: A critical review of studies from a systems-contextual perspective. *Clinical Psychology: Science and Practice, 17*(1), 1–30.

Beidas, R. S., Koerner, K., Weingardt, K. R., & Kendall, P. C. (2011). Training research: Practical recommendations for maximum impact. *Administration and Policy in Mental Health and Mental Health Services Research, 38*(4), 223–237.

Bekelman, J. E., Li, Y., & Gross, C. P. (2003). Scope and impact of financial conflicts of interest in biomedical research: A systematic review. *Journal of the American Medical Association, 289*, 454–465.

Beutler, L. E. (2000). David and Goliath: When empirical and clinical standards of practice meet. *American Psychologist, 55*, 997–1007.

Bischoff, R. J., Springer, P. R., Felix, D. S., & Hollist, C. S. (2011). Find the heart of medical family therapy: A content analysis of medical family therapy casebook articles. *Families, Systems, and Health, 29*, 184–196.

Bisson, J., & Andrew, M. (2009). Psychological treatment of posttraumatic stress disorder (PTSD). *Cochrane Database of Systematic Reviews, 4.* Retrieved from the Cochrane Library database.

Bohart, A. C., O'Hara, M., & Leitner, L. M. (1998). Empirically violated treatments: Disenfranchisement of humanistic and other psychotherapies. *Psychotherapy Research, 8*(2), 141–157.

Bollen, J., Van de Sompel, H., Hagberg, A., & Chute, R. (2009). A principal component analysis of 39 scientific impact measures. *PLoS ONE, 4*(6), e6022.

Bordin, E. S. (1979). The generalizability of the psychoanalytic concept of the working alliance. *Psychotherapy: Theory, Research, and Practice, 16,* 252–260.

Bordons, M., Fernández, M. T., & Gómez, I. (2002). Advantages and limitations in the use of impact factor measures for the assessment of research performance in a peripheral country. *Scientometrics, 53,* 195–206.

Bowser, B. P., Word, C. O., Stanton, M. D., & Coleman, S. B. (2003). Death in the family and HIV risk-taking among intravenous drug users. *Family Process, 42,* 291–304.

Bradburn, N., Sudman, S., & Wansink, B. (2004). *Asking questions: The definitive guide to questionnaire design—for market research, political polls, and social and health questionnaires* (rev. ed.). San Francisco: Jossey-Bass.

Bradley, B., & Furrow, J. L. (2004). Toward a mini-theory of the blamer softener event: Tracking the moment-to-moment process. *Journal of Marital and Family Therapy, 30,* 233–246.

Bradley, B., & Johnson, S. M. (2005). Task analysis of couple and family change events. In D. H. Sprenkle & F. P. Piercy (Eds.), *Research methods in family therapy* (2nd ed., pp. 254–271). New York: Guilford Press.

Bremer, R. W., Scholle, S. H., Keyser, D., Knox Houtsinger, J. V., & Pincus, H. A. (2008). Pay for performance in behavioral health. *Psychiatric Services, 59*(12), 1419–1429.

Breunlin, D. C., Pinsof, W., & Russell, W. P. (2011). Integrative Problem-Centered Metaframeworks Therapy I: Core concepts and hypothesizing. *Family Process, 50,* 293–313.

Brinkmeyer, M. Y., & Eyberg, S. M. (2003). Parent–child interaction therapy for oppositional children. In A. E. Kazdin & J. R. Weisz (Eds.), *Evidence-based psychotherapies for children and adolescents* (pp. 204–223). New York: Guilford Press.

Buckingham, J., Fisher, B., & Saunders, D. (2012). *Evidence Based Medicine Toolkit.* Retrieved September 1, 2012, from *www.ebm.med.ualberta.ca.*

Burke, D., & Phillips, L. H. (2012). Is the "impact factor" a valid measure of the impact of research published in *Clinical Neurophysiology* and *Muscle & Nerve? Clinical Neurophysiology, 123,* 1687–1690.

Burlingame, G. M., Wells, M. G., Lambert, M. J., & Cox, J. C. (2004). Youth Outcome Questionnaire (Y-OQ). In M. E. Maruish (Ed.), *The use of psychological testing for treatment planning and outcome assessment* (3rd ed., Vol. 2, pp. 235–274). Mahwah, NJ: Erlbaum.

Callaway, E. (2011). Massive fraud uncovered in work by social psychologist. *Nature,*

479, 15. Retrieved March 23, 2012, from *www.nature.com/news/2011/111101/ full/479015a.html.*

Carr, A. (2012). *Family therapy: Concepts, process, and practice* (3rd ed.). West Sussex, UK: Wiley.

Carroll, J. S., & Doherty, W. J. (2003). Evaluating the effectiveness of premarital prevention programs: A meta-analytic review of outcome research. *Family Relations, 52,* 105–118.

Center for Marriage and Family. (1999). *Ministry to interchurch marriages: A national study.* Omaha, NE: Creighton University.

Centers for Disease Control and Prevention. (2011). *U.S. Public Health Service syphilis study at Tuskegee: The Tuskegee timeline.* Retrieved April 17, 2012, from *www.cdc.gov/tuskegee/timeline.htm.*

Chambless, D. L., & Hollon, S. (1998). Defining empirically supported therapies. *Journal of Consulting and Clinical Psychology, 66,* 7–18.

Chambless, D. L., Sanderson, W. C., Shoham, V., Johnson, S. B., Pope, K. S., Crits-Christoph, P., . . . McCurry, S. (1996). An update on empirically validated treatments. *The Clinical Psychologist, 49*(2), 5–18.

Charles, C., Gafni, A., & Whelan, T. (1997). Shared decision making in the medical encounter: What does it mean? (or it takes at least two to tango). *Social Science and Medicine, 44*(5), 681–692.

Chase, R. M., & Eyberg, S. M. (2008). Clinical presentation and treatment outcome for children with comorbid externalizing and internalizing symptoms. *Anxiety Disorders, 22,* 273–282.

Chenail, R. J., St. George, S., Wulff, D., Duffy, M., Scott, K. W., & Tomm, K. (2012). Clients' relational conceptions of conjoint couples and family therapy quality: A grounded formal theory. *Journal of Marital and Family Therapy, 38,* 241–264.

Cohen, J. (1988). *Statistical power analysis for behavior sciences* (2nd ed.). Hillsdale, NJ: Erlbaum.

Cohen, S. (2004). Social relationships and health. *American Psychologist, 59,* 676–684.

Cohen, S., Doyle, W. J., Skoner, D. P., Rabin, B. S., & Gwaltney, J. M., Jr. (1997). Social ties and susceptibility to the common cold. *Journal of the American Medical Association, 277,* 1940–1944.

Collins, L., & Ladd, R. (2007). EBBP search for evidence module. In *Evidence-based behavioral practice.* Retrieved July 18, 2012, from *www.ebbp.org/training.html.*

Committee on Quality Health Care in America. (2001). *Crossing the quality chasm: A new health system for the 21st century.* Washington, DC: Institute of Medicine, National Academies Press. Retrieved from *www.nap.edu/books/0309072808/ html.*

Council for Training in Evidence-Based Behavioral Practice. (2008, July). Definition and competencies for evidence-based behavioral practice (EBBP). In *Evidence-Based Behavioral Practice.* Retrieved April 15, 2012, from *www.ebbp.org/ documents/EBBP_Competencies.pdf.*

Couper, M. P., Singer, E., Levin, C. A., Fowler, F. J., Fagerlin, A., & Zikmund-

Fisher, B. J. (2010). Use of the Internet and ratings of information sources for medical decisions: Results from the DECISIONS survey. *Medical Decision Making*, 30(5), 106S–114S.

Cozby, C. Z. (2004). *Methods in behavioral research* (8th ed.). New York: McGraw-Hill.

Crane, D. R., & Hafen, M. (2002). Meeting the needs of evidence-based practice in family therapy: Developing the scientist–practitioner model. *Journal of Family Therapy*, 24, 113–124.

Cummings, N. A. (2006). Psychology, the stalwart profession, faces new challenges and opportunities. *Professional Psychology: Research and Practice*, 37(6), 598–605.

Dahl, C. M., & Boss, P. (2005). The use of phenomenology in family therapy research. In D. H. Sprenkle & F. P. Piercy (Eds.), *Research methods in family therapy* (2nd ed., pp. 63–84). New York: Guilford Press.

Damschroder, L. J., Aron, D. C., Keith, R. E., Kirsh, S. R., Alexander, J. A., & Lowery, J. C. (2009, August 7). Fostering implementation of health services research findings into practice: A consolidated framework for advancing implementation science. *Implementation Science*, 4, 50.

Dattilio, F. M., Piercy, F. P., & Davis, S. D. (2014). The divide between "evidence-based" approaches and practitioners of traditional theories of family therapy. *Journal of Marital and Family Therapy*, 40, 5–16.

Davidson, K. W., Trudeau, K. J., Ockene, J. K., Orleans, C. T., & Kaplan, R. M. (2004). A primer on current evidence-based review systems and their implication for behavioral medicine. *Annals of Behavioral Medicine*, 28(3), 226–238.

Diamond, G. M., Liddle, H. A., Hogue, A., & Dakof, G. A. (1999). Alliance-building interventions with adolescents in family therapy: A process study. *Psychotherapy*, 36, 355–368.

Dimidjian, S., Martell, C. R., & Christensen, A. (2008). Integrative behavioral couple therapy. In A. S. Gurman (Ed.), *Clinical handbook of couple therapy* (4th ed., pp. 73–103). New York: Guilford Press.

Drury, V., Francis, K., & Chapman, Y. (2007). Taming the rescuer: The therapeutic nature of qualitative research interviews. *International Journal of Nursing Practice*, 13, 383–384.

Duncan, B. L., Miller, S. D., & Sparks, J. (2004). *The heroic client: A revolutionary way to improve effectiveness through client-directed, outcome-informed therapy* (2nd ed.). San Francisco: Jossey-Bass.

Duncan, B. L., & Miller, S. D. (2008). *The Outcome and Session Rating Scales: The revised administration and scoring manual, including the Child Outcome Rating Scale*. Chicago: Institute for the Study of Therapeutic Change.

Echevarria-Doan, S., & Tubbs, C. Y. (2005). Let's get grounded: Family therapy research and grounded theory. In D. H. Sprenkle & F. P. Piercy (Eds.), *Research methods in family therapy* (2nd ed., pp. 41–62). New York: Guilford Press.

Edwards, K. A. (2008). Informed consent. In *Ethics in medicine*. Retrieved June 12, 2012, from *http://depts.washington.edu/bioethx/topics/consent.html*.

Edwards, T. M., Patterson, J., Scherger, J., & Vakili, S. (in press). Policy and practice: A primer on the past, present, and future of health care reform in the United States. In J. Hodgson, A. Lamson, T. Mendenhall, & R. Crane (Eds). *Medical family therapy: Advanced applications.* New York: Springer.

Edwards, T. M., Patterson, J., Vakili, S., & Scherger, J. (2012). Health care policy in the United States: A primer for medical family therapists. *Contemporary Family Therapy: An International Journal, 34,* 217–227.

Eijkenaar, F. (2013). Key issues in the design of pay for performance programs. *European Journal of Health Economics, 14*(1), 117–131.

Eisler, I., Dare, C., Hodes, M., Russell, G., Dodge, E., & le Grange, D. (2000). Family therapy for adolescent anorexia nervosa: The results of a controlled comparison of two family interventions. *Journal of Child Psychology and Psychiatry, 41,* 727–736.

Eisler, I., Simic, M., Russell, G. F. M., & Dare, C. (2007). A randomised controlled treatment trial of two forms of family therapy in adolescent anorexia nervosa: A 5-year follow-up. *Journal of Child Psychology and Psychiatry, 48,* 552–560.

Elliot, R. (2008). Research on client experiences of therapy: Introduction to the special section. *Psychotherapy Research, 18,* 239–242.

Elliott, R., & James, E. (1989). Varieties of client experience in psychotherapy: An analysis of the literature. *Clinical Psychology Review, 9,* 443–468.

Epstein, N., & Baucom, D. H. (2002). *Enhanced cognitive-behavioral couple therapy for couples: A contextual approach.* Washington, DC: American Psychological Association.

Epstein, N. B., Baldwin, L. M., & Bishop, D. S. (1983). The McMaster Family Assessment Device. *Journal of Marital and Family Therapy, 9,* 171–180.

Field, A., & Cottrell, D. (2011). Eye movement desensitization and reprocessing as a therapeutic intervention for traumatized children and adolescents: A systematic review of the evidence for family therapists. *Journal of Family Therapy, 33,* 374–388.

Fisher, C. B., & Oransky, M. (2008). Informed consent to psychotherapy: Protecting the dignity and respecting the autonomy of patients. *Journal of Clinical Psychology, 64*(5), 576–588.

Flori, D. E. (1989). The prevalence of later life family concerns in the marriage and family therapy journal literature (1976–1985): A content analysis. *Journal of Marital and Family Therapy, 15,* 289–297.

Forgatch, M. S., & Chamberlain, P. (1982). The Therapist Behavior Code. Unpublished instrument and technical report, Oregon Social Learning Center, Eugene, OR.

Fowler, F. J., Levin, C. A., & Sepucha, K. R. (2011). Informing and involving patients to improve the quality of medical decisions. *Health Affairs, 30*(4), 699–706.

Franklin, M. E., & DeRubeis, R. J. (2006). Efficacious laboratory-validated treatments are generally transportable to clinical practice. In J. C. Norcross & L. E. Beutler (Eds.), *Evidence-based practices in mental health: Debate and dialogue on the fundamental questions* (pp. 375–383). Washington, DC: American Psychological Association.

Friedlander, M. (2009). Addressing systemic challenges in couple and family therapy research: Introduction to the special section. *Psychotherapy Research, 19,* 129–132.

Friedlander, M. L., Escudero, V., Horvath, A. O., Heatherington, L., Cabero, A., & Martens, M. P. (2006). System for observing family therapy alliances: A tool for research and practice. *Journal of Counseling Psychology, 53,* 214–224.

Fritz, J. M., & Cleland, J. (2003). Effectiveness versus efficacy: More than a debate over language. *Journal of Orthopaedic & Sports Physical Therapy, 33,* 163–165.

Fruzetti, A. E., & Fantozzi, B. (2008). Couple therapy and the treatment of borderline personality and related disorders. In A. S. Gurman (Ed.), *Clincial handbook of couple therapy* (4th ed., pp. 567–590). New York: Guilford Press.

Gale, J. (1996). Conversation analyses: Studying the construction of therapeutic realities. In D. H. Sprenkle & S. M. Moon (Eds.), *Research methods in family therapy* (pp. 107–124). New York: Guilford Press.

Garfield, S. L. (1996). Some problems associated with "validated" forms of psychotherapy. *Clinical Psychology: Science & Practice, 3,* 218–229.

Garland, A. F., Brookman-Frazee, L., Hurlburt, M. S., Accurso, E. C., Zoffness, R. J., Haine-Schlagel, R., & Ganger, W. (2010). Mental health care for children with disruptive behavior problems: A view inside the therapists' offices. *Psychiatric Services, 61,* 788–795.

Gibbs, L. E. (2003). *Evidence-based practice for the helping professions: A practical guide with integrated multimedia.* Pacific Grove, CA: Brooks/Cole-Thomson Learning.

Glaser, R., Kiecolt-Glaser, J. K., Marucha, P. T., MacCallum, R. C., Laskowski, B. F., & Malarkey, W. B. (1999). Stress-related changes in proinflammatory cytokine production in wounds. *Archives of General Psychiatry, 56,* 450–456.

Gludd, L. L., Sørensen, T. I., Gøtzsche, P. C., & Gluud, C. (2005). The journal impact factor as a predictor of trial quality and outcomes: Cohort study of hepatobiliary randomized clinical trials. *American Journal of Gastroenterology, 100*(11), 2431–2435.

Goleman, D. (2007). *Social intelligence: The new science of human relationships.* New York: Bantam.

Gordon, K. C., Baucom, D. H., & Snyder, D. K. (2004). An integrative intervention for promoting recovery from extramarital affairs. *Journal of Marital and Family Therapy, 30,* 213–231.

Gordon, K. C., Baucom, D. H., Snyder, D. K., & Dixon, L. J. (2008). Couple therapy and the treatment of affairs. In A. S. Gurman (Ed.), *Clinical handbook of couple therapy* (4th ed., pp. 429–458). New York: Guilford Press.

Gottman, J. M. (1993). *What predicts divorce?: The relationship between marital processes and marital outcomes.* Hillsdale, NJ: Erlbaum.

Gottman, J. M., & Gottman, J. S. (2008). Gottman Method Couple Therapy. In A. S. Gurman (Ed.), *Clinical handbook of couple therapy* (4th ed., pp. 138–164). New York: Guilford Press.

Greenhalgh, T. (2010). *How to read a paper: The basics of evidence-based medicine* (4th ed.). West Sussex, UK: BMJ Publishing Group.

Gurman, A. S., & Kniskern, D. P. (1981). Family therapy process research: Knowns and unknowns. In A. S. Gurman & D. P. Kniskern (Eds.), *Handbook of family therapy* (pp. 742–775). New York: Brunner/Mazel.

Guyatt, G., & Rennie, D. (1993). Users' guides to the medical literature. *Journal of the American Medical Association, 270*(17), 2096–2097.

Guyatt, G., Rennie, D., Meade, M. O., & Cook, D. J. (Eds.). (2008). *Users' guides to the medical literature: A manual evidence-based clinical practice* (2nd ed.). New York: McGraw-Hill.

Hall, C. A., & Sandberg, J. G. (2012). "We shall overcome": A qualitative exploratory study of the experiences of African Americans who overcame barriers to engage in family therapy. *American Journal of Family Therapy, 40,* 445–458.

Hartley, D., & Strupp, H. (1983). The therapeutic alliance: Its relationship to outcome in brief psychotherapy. In J. Masling (Ed.), *Empirical studies of psychoanalytic theories* (pp. 1–27). Hillsdale, NJ: Erlbaum.

Hatcher, R. L., & Gillaspy, J. A. (2006). Development and validation of a revised short version of the Working Alliance Inventory. *Psychotherapy Research, 16,* 12–25.

Heatherington, L., & Friedlander, M. L. (1990). Couple and family therapy alliance scales: Empirical considerations. *Journal of Marital and Family Therapy, 16,* 299–306.

Henggeler, S. W., & Sheidow, A. J. (2003). Conduct disorder and delinquency. *Journal of Marital and Family Therapy, 29,* 505–522.

Henggeler, S. W., & Sheidow, A. J. (2012). Empirically supported family-based treatments for conduct disorder and delinquency in adolescents. *Journal of Marital and Family Therapy, 38,* 30–58.

Herschell, A. D., Kolko, D. J., Baumann, B. L., & Davis, A. C. (2010). The role of therapist training in the implementation of psychosocial treatments: A review and critique with recommendations. *Clinical Psychology Review, 30,* 448–466.

Hodgson, J. L., Johnson, L. N., Ketring, S. A., Wampler, R. S., & Lamson, A. L. (2005). Integrating research and clinical training in marriage and family therapy training programs. *Journal of Marital and Family Therapy, 31,* 75–88.

Horvath, A. O. (1994). Empirical validation of Bordin's pantheoretical model of the alliance: The Working Alliance Inventory perspective. In A. O. Horvath & L. S. Greenberg (Eds.), *The working alliance: Theory, research, and practice* (pp. 109–128). New York: Wiley.

Horvath, A. O., & Greenberg, L. S. (1986). The development of the Working Alliance Inventory. In L. S. Greenberg & W. M. Pinsof (Eds.), *The psychotherapeutic process: A research handbook* (pp. 529–556). New York: Guilford Press.

Horvath, A. O., & Greenberg, L. S. (1989). Development and validation of the Working Alliance Inventory. *Journal of Counseling Psychology, 36,* 223–233.

Howard, K. I., Kopte, S. M., Krause, M. S., & Orlinsky, D. E. (1986). The dose-effect relationship in psychotherapy. *American Psychologist, 41,* 159–164.

Howard, K. I., Lueger, R. J., Maling, M. S., & Martinovich, Z. (1993). A phase model of psychotherapy outcome: Causal mediation of change. *Journal of Consulting and Clinical Psychology, 61,* 678–685.

Howard, K. I., Moras, K., Brill, P. L., Martinovich, Z., & Lutz, W. (1996). Evaluation of psychotherapy: Efficacy, effectiveness, and patient progress. *American Psychologist, 51,* 1059–1064.

Jager, K. B., Bak, J., Barber, A., Bozek, K., Bocknek, E. L., & Weir, G. (2009). Qualitative inquiry and family therapist identity construction through community-based child welfare practice. *Journal of Feminist Family Therapy, 21,* 39–57.

Jewell, J. D., & Stark, K. D. (2003). Comparing family environments of adolescents with conduct disorder or depression. *Journal of Child and Family Studies, 12*(1), 77–89.

John, A., & Montgomery, D. (2012). Socialization goals of first-generation immigrant Indian parents: A Q-methodological study. *Asian American Journal of Psychology, 3,* 299–312.

Johnson, L. N., Wright, D. W., & Ketring, S. A. (2002). The therapeutic alliance in home-based family therapy: Is it predictive of outcome? *Journal of Marital and Family Therapy, 28,* 93–102.

Johnson, S. M. (2003). The revolution in couple therapy: A practitioner–scientist perspective. *Journal of Marital and Family Therapy, 29,* 365–384.

Johnson, S. M. (2004). *The practice of emotionally focused couple therapy: Creating connection* (2nd ed.). New York: Brunner-Routledge.

Johnson, S. M., & Greenberg, L. S. (1988). Relating process to outcome in marital therapy. *Journal of Marital and Family Therapy, 14,* 175–183.

Johnson, S. M., Hunsley, J., Greenberg, L., & Schindler, D. (1999). Emotionally focused couples therapy: Status and challenges. *Clinical Psychology: Science and Practice, 6,* 67–79.

Johnson, S. M., Makinen, M., & Millikin, J. (2001). Attachment injuries in couple relationships: A new perspective on impasses in couple therapy. *Journal of Marital and Family Therapy, 27,* 145–155.

Jose, A., O'Leary, K. D., & Moyer, A. (2010). Does premarital cohabitation predict subsequent marital stability and marital quality?: A meta-analysis. *Journal of Marriage and the Family, 72,* 105–116.

Kamalabadi, M. J., Ahmadi, S. A., Etemadi, O., Fatehizadeh, M., Baharami, F., & Firoozabadi, A. (2012). A study of the effect of couple dialectical behavioral therapy on symptoms and quality of marital relationships and mental health of Iranian borderline personality couples: A controlled trial. *Interdisciplinary Journal of Contemporary Research in Business, 3*(9), 1480–1487.

Karam, E. A., & Sprenkle, D. H. (2010). The research-informed clinician: A guide to training the next-generation MFT. *Journal of Marital and Family Therapy, 36,* 307–319.

Kazdin, A. E. (2005). *Parent management training treatment for oppositional, aggressive, and antisocial behavior in children and adolescents.* New York: Oxford University Press.

Keitner, G. I., Heru, A. M., & Glick, I. D. (2010). *Clinical manual of couples and family therapy.* Washington, DC: American Psychiatric Publishing, Inc.

Keitner, G. I., Ryan, C. E., Miller, J. W., & Norman, W. H. (1992). Recovery and major depression: Factors associated with 12-month outcome. *American Journal of Psychiatry, 149,* 93–99.

Kelley, M. L., & Fals-Stewart, W. (2002). Couples versus individual-based therapy for alcoholism and drug abuse: Effects on children's psychosocial functioning. *Journal of Consulting and Clinical Psychology, 70*, 417–427.

Kent, D., & Hayward, R. (2007). When averages hide individual differences in clinical trials. *American Scientist, 95*, 60–72.

Kiecolt-Glaser, J. K, Glaser, R., & Malarkey, W. B. (1999). Marital stress: Immunologic, neuroendocrine, and autonomic correlates. *Annals of the New York Academy of Sciences, 840*, 656–663.

Kroenke, K., Spitzer, R. L., & Williams, J. B. W. (2001). The PHQ-9: Validity of a brief depression measure. *Journal of General Internal Medicine, 16*(9), 606–613.

Kuehl, B. P., Newfield, N. A., & Joanning, H. (1990). A client-based description of family therapy. *Journal of Family Psychology, 3*, 310–321.

Kurtzman, H., & Bufka, L. (2011). APA moves forward on developing clinical treatment guidelines: Steering committee designs, policies, and procedures for new APA activity. In *Practice Central*. Retrieved April 19, 2012, from *www.apapracticecentral.org/update/2011/07–14/clinical-treatment.aspx*.

Lambert, M. J. (2013). *Bergin and Garfield's handbook of psychotherapy and behavior change* (6th ed.). Hoboken, NJ: John Wiley.

Lambert, M. J., Bailey, R. J., Kimball, K., Shimokawa, K., Harmon, S. C., & Slade, K. (2007). *Clinical support tools manual, brief version-40*. Salt Lake City: OQ Measures LLC.

Lambert, M. J., Morton, J. J., Hatfield, D., Harmon, C., Hamilton, S., Reid, R. C., & Burlingame, G. M. (2004). *Administration and scoring manual for the Outcome Questionnaire, 45*. Salt Lake City, UT: OQ Measures.

Lambert, M. J., & Shimokawa, K. (2011). Collecting client feedback. *Psychotherapy, 48*, 72–79.

Lambert, M. J., Whipple, J., Smart, D., Vermeersch, D., Nielsen, S., & Hawkins, E. (2001). The effects of providing therapists with feedback on patient progress during psychotherapy: Are outcomes enhanced? *Psychotherapy Research, 11*(1), 49–68.

Lambert-Shute, J., & Fruhauf, C. A. (2011). Aging issues: Unanswered questions in marital and family therapy literature. *Journal of Marital and Family Therapy, 37*, 27–36.

Lebow, J. (2006). *Research for the psychotherapist: From science to practice*. New York: Routledge.

Lebow, J. L., Chambers, A. L., Christensen, A., & Johnson, S. M. (2012). Research on the treatment of couple distress. *Journal of Marital and Family Therapy, 38*, 145–168.

Leffler, J. M., Jackson, Y., West, A. E., McCarty, C. A., & Atkins, M. S. (2012). Training in evidence-based practice across the professional continuum. *Professional Psychology: Research and Practice, 44*(1), 20–28.

Légaré, F., Bekker, H., Desroches, S., Drolet, R., Politi, M., Stacey, D., . . . Sullivan, M. D. (2011). How can continuing professional development better promote shared decision making? Perspectives from an international collaboration. *Implementation Science, 6*, 68.

Légaré, F., Elwyn, G., Fishbein, M., Frémont, P., Frosch, D., Gagnon, M., . . . vander Weijden, T. (2008). Translating shared decision making into health care clinical practices: Proof of concepts. *Implementation Science, 3,* 2.

Levant, R. F., & Hasan, N. T. (2008). Evidence-based practice in psychology. *Professional Psychology: Research and Practice, 39*(6), 658–662.

Levinson, W., Kao, A., Kuby, A., & Thisted, R. A. (2005). Not all patients want to participate in decision making. *Journal of General Internal Medicine, 20,* 531–535.

Liddle, H. A. (1991). Empirical values and the culture of family therapy. *Journal of Marital and Family Therapy, 17,* 327–348.

Lokker, C., Haynes, R. B., Chu, R., McKibbon, K. A., Wilczynski, N. L., & Walter, S. D. (2012). How well are journal and clinical article characteristics associated with the journal impact factor? A retrospective cohort study. *Journal of the Medical Library Association, 100*(1), 28–33.

Lubell, J. (2013). Mental health minimum benefits bolstered. *American Medical News, 56*(5), 1–4.

Lucksted, A., McFarlane, W., Downing, D., Dixon, L., & Adams, C. (2012). Recent development in family psychoeducation as an evidence-based practice. *Journal of Marital and Family Therapy, 38,* 101–121.

Lucock, M. P., Hall, P., & Noble, R. (2006). A survey of influences on the practice of psychotherapists and clinical psychologists in the UK. *Clinical Psychology & Psychotherapy, 13,* 123–130.

Luebbe, A., Radcliffe, A., Callands, T., Green, D., & Thorn, B. E. (2007). Evidence-based practice in psychology: Perceptions of graduate students in scientist-practitioner programs. *Journal of Clinical Psychology, 63*(7), 643–655.

Makinen, J. A., & Johnson, S. M. (2006). Resolving attachment injuries in couples using emotionally focused therapy: Steps toward forgiveness and reconciliation. *Journal of Consulting and Clinical Psychology, 74,* 1055–1064.

March, J., Silva, S., Petrycki, S., Curry, J., Wells, K., Fairbank, J., . . . the Treatment for Adolescents with Depression (2004). Fluoxetine, cognitive-behavioral therapy, and their combination for adolescents with depression: Treatment for Adolescents with Depression Study (TADS) randomized controlled trial. *Journal of the American Medical Association, 292*(7), 807–820.

Markoff, J. (2013, March 6). Unreported side effects of drugs are found using Internet search data. *New York Times.* Retrieved May 15, 2013, from *www.nytimes.com/2013/03/07/science/unreported-side-effects-of-drugs-found-using-internet-data-study-finds.html.*

Mathieu, E. (2010). The Internet and medical decision making: Can it replace the role of health care providers? *Medical Decision Making, 30*(5), 14S–16S.

McCoyd, J. L., & Shdaimah, C. S. (2007). Revisiting the benefits debate: Does qualitative social work research produce salubrious effects? *Social Work, 52,* 340–349.

McFarlane, W. R., Dixon, L., Lukens, E., & Lucksted, A. (2003). Family psychoeducation and schizophrenia: A review of the literature. *Journal of Marital and Family Therapy, 29,* 223–245.

Milgram, S. (1963). Behavioral study of obedience. *Journal of Abnormal and Social Psychology*, 67, 371–378.

Miller, S. D., Duncan, B. L., Brown, J., Sorrell, R., & Chalk, M. B. (2006). Using formal feedback to improve retention and outcome: Making ongoing, real-time assessment feasible. *Journal of Brief Therapy*, 5, 5–22.

Miller, S. D., Duncan, B. L., Brown, J., Sparks, J. A., & Claud, D. A. (2003). The outcome rating scale: A preliminary study of the reliability, validity, and feasibility of a brief visual analog measure. *Journal of Brief Therapy*, 2, 91–100.

Miller, S. D., Duncan, B. L., Sorrell, R., & Brown, G. S. (2005). The partners for change outcome system. *Journal of Clinical Psychology: In Session*, 61, 199–208.

Minuchin, S. (1974). *Families and family therapy*. Cambridge, MA: Harvard University Press.

Moher, D., Hopewell, S., Schulz, K. F., Montori, V., Gøtzsche, P. C., Devereaux, P. J., . . . Altman, D. G. (2010). CONSORT 2010 Explanation and Elaboration: Updated guidelines for reporting parallel group randomised trial. *British Medical Journal*, 340, c869. Retrieved April 1, 2013, from *www.bmj.com/content/340/bmj.c869*.

Murray, B. L. (2003). Qualitative research interviews: Therapeutic benefits for participants. *Journal of Psychiatric and Mental Health Nursing*, 10, 233–236.

Murrow, C., & Shi, L. (2010). The influence of cohabitation purposes on relationship quality: An examination of dimensions. *American Journal of Family Therapy*, 38, 397–412.

National Institute of Mental Health. (2012). NIMH: The 2012 Fiscal Year. In *National Institute of Mental Health: The President's Budget Request*. Retrieved July 2, 2012, from *www.nimh.nih.gov/about/budget/cj2012.pdf*.

Nelson, T. S., Chenail, R. J., Alexander, J. F., Crane, D. R., Johnson, S. M., & Schwallie, L. (2007). The development of core competencies for the practice of marriage and family therapy. *Journal of Marital and Family Therapy*, 33, 417–438.

Nelson, T. S., & Graves, T. (2011). Core competencies in advanced training: What supervisors say about graduate training. *Journal of Marital and Family Therapy*, 37, 429–451.

Norcross, J. (Ed.). (2011). *Psychotherapy relationships that work: Evidence-based responsiveness* (2nd ed.). New York: Oxford University Press.

Norcross, J. C., Beutler, L. E., & Levant, R. F. (2006). *Evidence-based practices in mental health: Debate and dialogue on the fundamental questions*. Washington, DC: American Psychological Association.

Norcross, J. C., & Lambert, M. J. (2011). Psychotherapy relationships that work II. *Psychotherapy*, 48, 4–8.

Norcross, J. C., & Wampold, B. E. (2011). Evidence-based therapy relationships: Research conclusions and clinical practices. *Psychotherapy*, 48, 98–102.

Nunez, N., Poole, D. A., & Memon, A. (2003). Psychology's two cultures revisited: Implications for the integration of science with practice. *Scientific Review of Mental Health Practice*, 2, 8–19.

O'Connor, E., Whitlock, E., & Spring, B. (2012). Introduction to Systematic

Reviews. Evidence-Based Behavioral-Practice Training Module. *www.ebbp. org/course_outlines/systematic_review*.

O'Farrell, T. J. (1993). *Treating alcohol problems: Marital and family interventions.* New York: Guilford Press.

O'Farrell, T. J., & Clements, K. (2012). Review of the outcome research on marital and family therapy for alcoholism. *Journal of Marital and Family Therapy, 38,* 122–144.

Olson, M. M., Russell, C. S., Higgins-Kessler, M., & Miller, R. B. (2002). Emotional processes following disclosure of an extramarital affair. *Journal of Marital and Family Therapy, 28,* 423–434.

Oxman, A. D., Sackett, D. L., & Guyatt, G. H. (1993). Users guide to medical literature: I. How to get started. *Journal of the American Medical Association, 207,* 2093–2095.

Pagoto, S., Spring, B., Coups, E., Mulvaney, S., Coutu, M., & Ozakinci, G. (2007). Barriers and facilitators of evidence-based practice perceived by behavioral science health professionals. *Journal of Clinical Psychology, 63*(7), 695–705.

Papernow, P. L. (2008). A clinician's view of "stepfamily architecture": Strategies for meeting the challenges. In J. Pryor (Ed.), *The international handbook of stepfamilies: Policy and practice in legal, research, and clinical environments* (pp. 423–454). Hoboken, NJ: John Wiley & Sons.

Patel, S., Bakken, S., & Ruland, C. (2008). Recent advances in shared decision making for mental health. *Current Opinion in Psychiatry, 21*(6), 606–612.

Patterson, J., Albala, A. A., McCahill, M. E., & Edwards, T. M. (2010). *The therapist's guide to psychopharmacology: Working with patients, families, and physicians to optimize care* (rev. ed.). New York: Guilford Press.

Patterson, J., Williams, L., Edwards, T. M., Chamow, L., & Grauf-Grounds, C. (2009). *Essential skills in family therapy: From the first interview to termination* (2nd ed.). New York: Guilford Press.

Patterson, J. E., Miller, R. B., Carnes, S., & Wilson, S. (2004). Evidence-based practice for marriage and family therapists. *Journal of Marital & Family Therapy, 30*(2), 183–195.

Paul, P. (2006, January 08). Getting sharp: Want a brainier baby? *Time.* Retrieved January 1, 2011, from *www.time.com/time/magazine/article/0,9171,1147180–4,00. html.*

Piercy, F. P., & Hertlein, K. M. (2005). Focus groups in family therapy research. In D. H. Sprenkle & F. P. Piercy (Eds.), *Research methods in family therapy* (2nd ed., pp. 85–99). New York: Guilford Press.

Pinsof, W. B., & Catherall, D. (1986). The integrative psychotherapy alliance: Family, couple, and individual scales. *Journal of Marital and Family Therapy, 12,* 137–151.

Pinsof, W. M., Zinbarg, R. E., Lebow, J. L., Knobloch-Fedders, L. M., Durbin, E., Chambers, A., . . . Friedman, G. (2009). Laying the foundation for progress research in family, couple, and individual therapy: The development and psychometric features of the initial systemic therapy inventory of change. *Psychotherapy Research, 19,* 143–156.

Pomerantz, A. M. (2005). Increasingly informed consent: Discussing distinct aspects of psychotherapy at different points in time. *Ethics & Behavior, 15,* 351–360.

Proulx, C. M., Helms, H. M., & Buehler, C. (2007). Marital quality and personal well-being: A meta-analysis. *Journal of Marriage and Family, 69,* 576–593.

Robbins, M. S., Liddle, H. A., Turner, C. W., Dakof, G. A., Alexander, J. F., & Kogan, S. M. (2006). Adolescent and parent therapeutic alliance as predictors of dropout in multidimensional family therapy. *Journal of Family Psychology, 20,* 108–116.

Robbins, M. S., Mayorga, C. C., Mitrani, V. B., Szapocznik, J., Turner, C. W., and Alexander, J. F. (2008). Adolescent and parent alliances with therapists in brief strategic family therapy with drug-using Hispanic adolescents. *Journal of Marital and Family Therapy, 34,* 316–328.

Rosen, G. M., & Davison, G. C. (2003). Psychology should list empirically supported principles of change (ESPs) and not credential trademark therapies or other treatment packages. *Behavior Modification, 27,* 300–312.

Rosenthal, M. B., & Frank, R. G. (2006). What is the empirical basis for paying for quality in healthcare? *Medical Care Research and Review, 63*(2), 135–157.

Rosser, S., Frede, S., Conrad, W., & Heaton, P. (2003). Development, implementation and evaluation of a pharmacist conducted screening program for depression. *Journal of the American Pharmacist Association, 53*(1) 22–29.

Rousmaniere, T. (Interviewer), & Lambert, M. (Interviewee). (2013). *Michael Lambert on preventing treatment failures (and why you're not as good as you think)* [Interview transcript]. Retrieved from *www.psychotherapy.net/interview/preventing-treatment-failures-lambert.*

Rowe, C. L. (2012). Family therapy for drug abuse: Review and updates, 2003–2010. *Journal of Marital and Family Therapy, 38,* 59–81.

Rubio, D. M., Schoenbaum, E. E., Lee, L. S., Schteingart, D. E., Marantz, P. R., Anderson, K. E., . . . Esposito, K. (2010). Defining translational research: Implications for training. *Academic Medicine, 85,* 470–475.

Rutledge, T., & Loh, C. (2004). Effect sizes and statistical testing in the determination of clinical significance in behavioral medicine research. *Annals of Behavioral Medicine, 27,* 138–145.

Sackett, D. L., Haynes, R. B., Tugwell, P., & Guyatt, G. H. (1991). *Clinical epidemiology: A basic science for clinical medicine* (2nd ed.). Philadelphia: Lippincott Williams & Wilkins.

Sackett, D. L., Straus, S., Richardson, S. W., Rosenberg, W., & Haynes, B. R. (2000). *Evidence-based medicine: How to practice and teach EBM* (2nd ed.). New York: Churchill Livingstone.

Saha, S., Saint, S., & Christakis, D. A. (2003). Impact factor: A valid measure of journal quality? *Journal of the Medical Library Association, 91*(1), 42–46.

Sandberg, J. G., Johnson, L. N., Robila, M., & Miller, R. B. (2002). Clinician identified barriers to clinical research. *Journal of Marital and Family Therapy, 28,* 61–67.

Satterfield, J. M., Springs, B., Brownson, R. C., Mullen, E. J., Newhouse, R. P.,

Walker, B. B., & Whitlock, E. P. (2010). Toward a transdisciplinary model of evidence-based practice. *Milbank Quarterly, 87*(2), 368–390.

Schulz, K. F., Altman, D. G., & Moher, D., for the CONSORT Group. (2010). CONSORT 2010 Statement: Updated guidelines for reporting parallel group randomised trials. *British Medical Journal, 340,* c332. Retrieved April 1, 2013, from *www.bmj.com/content/340/bmj.c332.*

Sepucha, K. R., Fagerlin, A., Couper, M. P., Levin, C. A., Singer, E., & Zikmund-Fisher, B. J. (2010). How does feeling informed relate to being informed?: The DECISIONS survey. *Medical Decision Making, 30,* 77–84.

Sexton, T., Gordon, K. C., Gurman, A., Lebow, J., Holtzworth-Munroe, A., & Johnson, S. (2011). Guidelines for classifying evidence-based treatments in couple and family therapy. *Family Process, 50,* 377–392.

Shadish, W. R., & Baldwin, S. A. (2003). Meta-analysis of MFT interventions. *Journal of Marital and Family Therapy, 29,* 547–570.

Shamai, M. (2003). Therapeutic effects of qualitative research: Reconstructing the experience of treatment as by-product of qualitative evaluation. *Social Service Review, 77,* 455–467.

Shelef, K., & Diamond, G. M. (2008). Short form of the revised Vanderbilt Therapeutic Alliance Scale: Development, reliability, and validity. *Psychotherapy Research, 18,* 433–443.

Shields, C., Wynne, L., McDaniel, S., & Gawinski, B. (1994). The marginalization of family therapy: A historical and continuing problem. *Journal of Marital and Family Therapy, 20,* 117–138.

Shields, C. G., Finley, M. A., Chawla, N., & Meadors, P. (2012). Couple and family interventions in health problems. *Journal of Marital and Family Therapy, 38,* 265–280.

Shirk, S. R., & Karver, M. (2003). Prediction of treatment outcome from relationship variables in child and adolescent therapy: A meta-analytic review. *Journal of Consulting and Clinical Psychology, 71,* 452–464.

Slesnick, N., & Prestopnik, J. L. (2005). Ecologically based family therapy outcome with substance abusing runaway adolescents. *Journal of Adolescence, 28,* 277–298.

Smith, R. (2005). Medical journals are an extension of the marketing arm of pharmaceutical companies. *PLoS Medicine, 2*(5): e138. Retrieved April 17, 2012, from *www.plosmedicine.org/article/info:doi/10.1371/journal.pmed.0020138.*

Snyder, D. K., Wills, R. M., & Grady-Fletcher, A. (1991). Long-term effectiveness of behavioral versus insight-oriented marital therapy: A 4-year follow-up study. *Journal of Consulting and Clinical Psychology, 59,* 138–141.

So, S. S., & LaGuardia, J. G. (2011). Matters of the heart: Patients' adjustment to life following a cardiac crisis. *Psychology & Health, 26,* 83–100.

Spanier, G. B. (1976). Measuring dyadic adjustment: New scales for assessing the quality of marriage and similar dyads. *Journal of Marriage and the Family, 38,* 15–28.

Sprenkle, D. H. (2004). *Effectiveness research in marriage and family therapy.* Alexandria, VA: American Association for Marriage and Family Therapy.

Sprenkle, D. H. (2012). Intervention research in couple and family therapy: A methodological and substantive review and an introduction to the special issue. *Journal of Marital and Family Therapy, 38*, 3–29.

Spring, B. (2007). Evidence-based practice in clinical psychology: What it is, why it matters; what you need to know. *Journal of Clinical Psychology, 63*(7), 611–631.

Spring, B., Abrantes, A. M., Kreslake, J. M., & Hitchcock, K. (2007). EBBP Process Module. In *Evidence-Based Behavioral Practice*. Retrieved April 15, 2012, from *www.ebbp.org/course_outlines/EBBP_Process*.

Stanley, S. M., Rhoades, G. K., & Markman, H. J. (2006). Sliding versus deciding: Inertia and the premarital cohabitation effect. *Family Relations, 55*, 499–509.

Stone, A. A. (1990). Law, science, and psychiatric malpractice: A response to Klerman's indictment of psychoanalytic psychiatry. *American Journal of Psychiatry, 147*, 419–427.

Strauss, A. L., & Corbin, J. (1998). *Basics of qualitative research: Techniques and procedures for developing grounded theory* (2nd ed.). Thousand Oaks, CA: Sage.

Sutherland, O., & Strong, T. (2011). Therapeutic collaboration: A conversation analysis of constructionist therapy. *Journal of Family Therapy, 33*, 256–278.

Tashiro, T., & Mortensen, L. (2006). Translational research: How social psychology can improve psychotherapy. *American Psychologist, 61*, 959–966.

Thomason, T. C. (2010). The trend toward evidence-based practice and the future of psychotherapy. *American Journal of Psychotherapy, 64*(1), 29–38.

Towle, A., & Godolphin, W. (1999). Framework for teaching and learning informed shared decision making. *British Medical Journal, 319*(7212), 766–771.

Tracey, T. J., & Kokotovic, A. M. (1989). Factor structure of the Working Alliance Inventory. *Psychological Assessment, 1*, 207–210.

Tryon, G. S., & Winograd, G. (2011). Goal consensus and collaboration. *Psychotherapy (Chicago, Ill), 48*(1), 50–57.

Tubbs, C. Y., & Burton, L. M. (2005). Bridging research: Using ethnography to inform clinical practice. In D. H. Sprenkle & F. P. Piercy (Eds.), *Research methods in family therapy* (2nd ed., pp. 136–154). New York: Guilford Press.

Turner, E. H., Matthews, A. M., Linardatos, E., Tell, R. A., & Rosenthal, R. (2008). Selective publication of antidepressant trials and its influence on apparent efficacy. *New England Journal of Medicine, 358*, 252–260.

University of Georgia, Institute for Evidence-Based Health Profession Education. (2012). Implications of the Affordable Care Act for evidence-based practice [Video file]. Retrieved from *www.youtube.com/watch?v=6lG_P_q3SSo&list=ECC9F945C67FE71151&index=18*.

Van Amburg, S. M., Barber, C. E., & Zimmerman, T. S. (1996). Aging and family therapy: Prevalence of aging issues and later family life concerns in marital and family therapy literature (1986–1993). *Journal of Marital and Family Therapy, 22*, 195–203.

Vucovich, L. A., Baker, J. B., & Smith, J. T. (2008). Analyzing the impact of an author's publications. *Journal of the Medical Library Association, 96*(1), 63–66.

Wade, W. A., Treat, T. A., & Stuart, G. L. (1998). Transporting an empirically supported treatment for panic disorder to a service clinic setting: A benchmarking strategy. *Journal of Consulting and Clinical Psychology, 66,* 231–239.

Walker, B. (2007). Novel tools and resources for evidence-based practice in psychology. *Journal of Clinical Psychology, 63*(7), 633–642.

Wampler, K. S., Reifman, A., & Serovich, J. M. (2005). Meta-analysis in family therapy research. In D. H. Sprenkle & F. P. Piercy (Eds.), *Research methods in family therapy* (2nd ed., pp. 318–338). New York: Guilford Press.

Weersing, V. R., & Weisz, J. R. (2002). Community clinic treatment of depressed youth: Benchmarking usual care against CBT clinical trials. *Journal of Consulting and Clinical Psychology, 70,* 299–310.

Westen, D. I. (2006a). Patients and treatments in clinical trials are not adequately representative of clinical practice. In J. C. Norcross & L. E. Beutler (Eds.), *Evidence-based practices in mental health: Debate and dialogue on the fundamental questions* (pp. 161–171). Washington, DC: American Psychological Association.

Westen, D. I. (2006b). Transporting laboratory-validated treatments to the community will not necessarily produce better outcomes. In J. C. Norcross & L. E. Beutler (Eds.), *Evidence-based practices in mental health: Debate and dialogue on the fundamental questions* (pp. 383–393). Washington, DC: American Psychological Association.

Westen, D. I., Novotny, C. M., & Thomas-Brenner, H. (2004). The empirical status of empirically supported psychotherapies: Assumptions, findings, and reporting in controlled trials. *Psychological Bulletin, 130,* 631–663.

Whisman, M. A. (2001). The association between depression and marital dissatisfaction. In S. R. H. Beach (Ed.), *Marital and family processes in depression* (pp. 3–24). Washington, DC: American Psychological Association.

Whisman, M. A., & Ubelacker, L. A. (2006). Impairment and distress associated with relationship discord in a national sample of married and cohabiting adults. *Journal of Family Psychology, 20,* 369–377.

Whitton, S. W., Nicholson, J. M., & Markman, H. J. (2008). Research on interventions for stepfamily couples: The state of the field. In J. Pryor (Ed.), *The international handbook of stepfamilies: Policy and practice in legal, research, and clinical environments* (pp. 455–484). Hoboken, NJ: John Wiley & Sons.

Williams, L., Edwards, T. M., Patterson, J., & Chamow, L. (2011). *Essential assessment skills for couple and family therapists.* New York: Guilford Press.

Williams, L., & Jurich, J. (1995). Predicting marital success after five years: Assessing the predictive validity of FOCCUS. *Journal of Marital and Family Therapy, 21,* 141–153.

Williams, L. M. (1995). The impact of stress on marital quality: A stress–vulnerability theory. *Contemporary Family Therapy, 17,* 217–227.

Williams, L. M., & Dombeck, H. J. (1999). To speak or not to speak: Guidelines for self-disclosure in supervision. In R. E. Lee & S. Emerson (Eds.), *The eclectic trainer* (pp. 22–30). Iowa City, IA: Geist & Russell.

Williams, L. M., & Lawler, M. G. (2000). The challenges and rewards of interchurch marriages: A qualitative study. *Journal of Psychology and Christianity, 19,* 205–218.

Williams, L. M., Patterson, J., & Miller R. B. (2006). Panning for gold: A clinician's guide to using research. *Journal of Marital and Family Therapy, 32,* 17–32.

Woolf, S. H. (2008). The meaning of translational research and why it matters. *Journal of the American Medical Association, 299*(2), 211–213.

World Health Organization. (2010). *mhGAP intervention guide for mental, neurological and substance abuse disorders in non-specialized health settings.* Retrieved September 29, 2013, from *http://whqlibdoc.who.int/publications/2010/9789241548069_eng.pdf.*

Yue, W., Wilson, C. S., & Boller, F. (2007). Peer assessment of journal quality in clinical neurology. *Journal of the Medical Library Association, 95*(1), 70–76.

Index

Page numbers followed by *f*, *t*, or *n* indicate a figure, a table, or a note; numbers in bold indicate glossary entries.